Ginseng - Modern Aspects of the Famed Traditional Medicine

Edited by Christophe Hano
and Jen-Tsung Chen

Published in London, United Kingdom

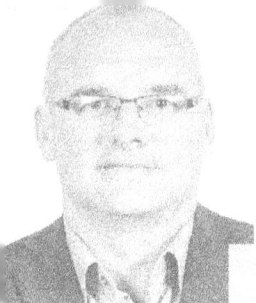
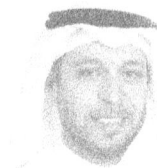
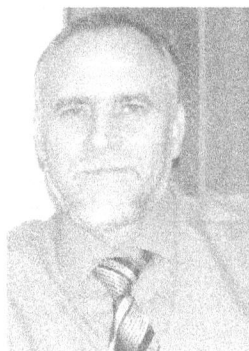
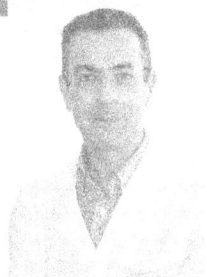
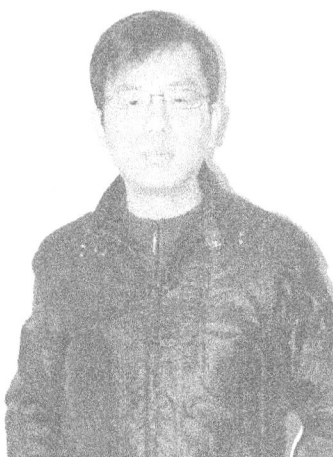
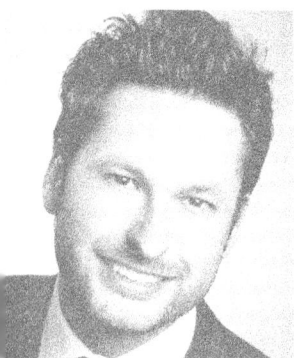
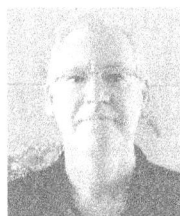

IntechOpen

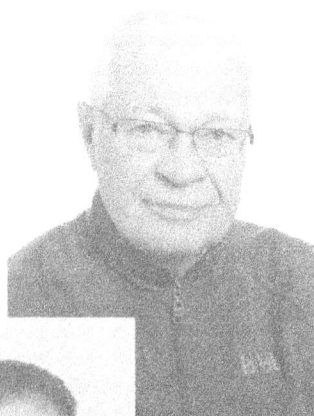
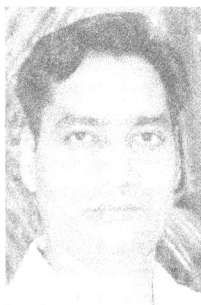
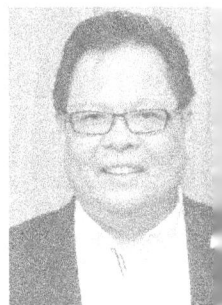
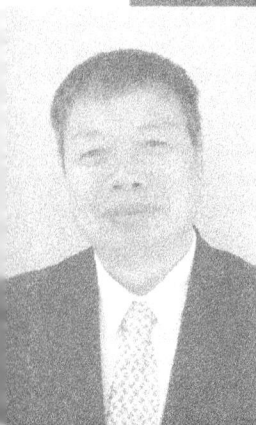
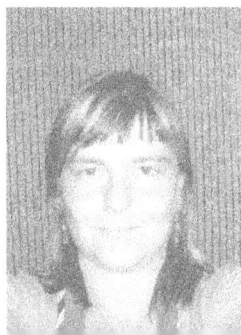
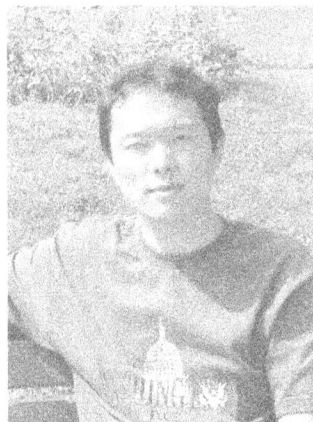

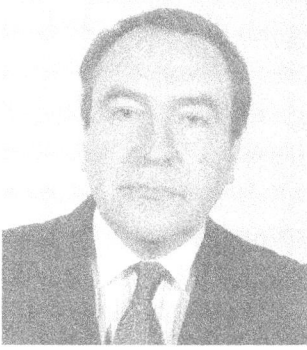

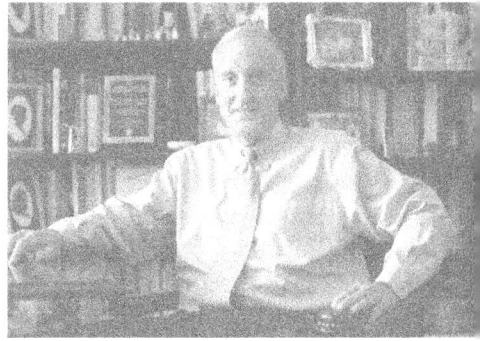

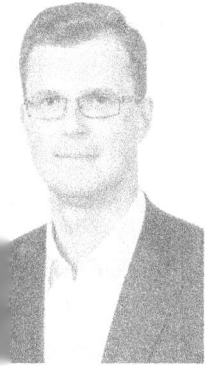

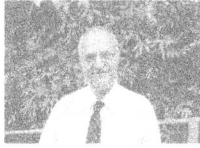

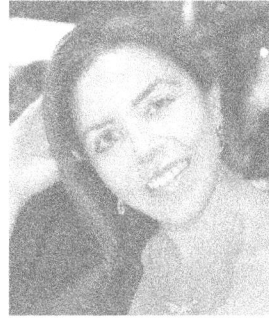

Supporting open minds since 2005

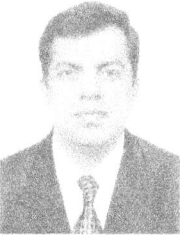

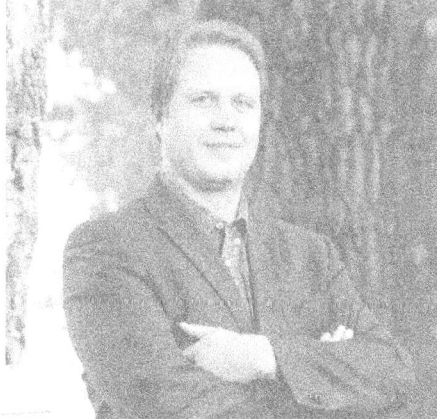

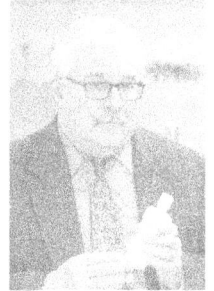

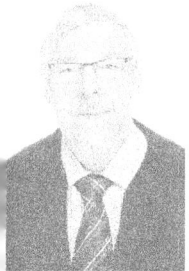

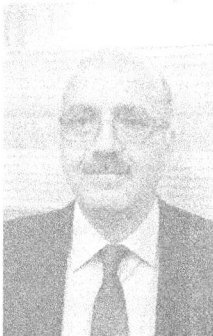

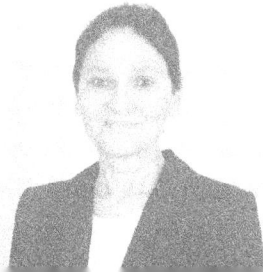

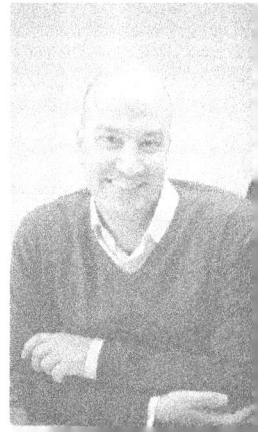

Ginseng - Modern Aspects of the Famed Traditional Medicine
http://dx.doi.org/10.5772/intechopen.92913
Edited by Christophe Hano and Jen-Tsung Chen

Contributors
Dimple Sethi Chopra, Abhishek Gupta, Dhandeep Singh, Nirmal Singh, Shuchi Dave Mehta, Priyanka
Rathore, Gopal Rai, Toluwase Hezekiah Fatoki, Mercedes De Mirecki-Garrido, Francisco Jimenez-
Acosta, Ruymán Santana-Farré, Noelia Guedes-Hernandez, Dionisio L. Lorenzo-Villegas, Christophe
F.E. Hano, Duangjai Tungmunnithum, Samantha Drouet, Mohamed Addi, Saikat Gantait, Jen-Tsung Chen

Notice
Statements and opinions expressed in the chapters are these of the individual contributors and not
necessarily those of the editors or publisher. No responsibility is accepted for the accuracy of
information contained in the published chapters. The publisher assumes no responsibility for any
damage or injury to persons or property arising out of the use of any materials, instructions, methods
or ideas contained in the book.

First published in London, United Kingdom, 2022 by IntechOpen
IntechOpen is the global imprint of INTECHOPEN LIMITED, registered in England and Wales,
registration number: 11086078, 5 Princes Gate Court, London, SW7 2QJ, United Kingdom
Printed in Croatia

British Library Cataloguing-in-Publication Data
A catalogue record for this book is available from the British Library

Additional hard and PDF copies can be obtained from orders@intechopen.com

Ginseng - Modern Aspects of the Famed Traditional Medicine
Edited by Christophe Hano and Jen-Tsung Chen
p. cm.
Print ISBN 978-1-83969-056-3
Online ISBN 978-1-83969-057-0
eBook (PDF) ISBN 978-1-83969-058-7

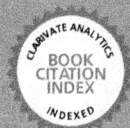

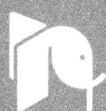

Meet the editors

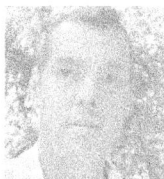

Dr. Christophe Hano is a phytochemist and an assistant professor at the University of Orléans, France. His research interests include plant specialized metabolism and plant biotechnology for nutraceutical, medicinal, and cosmeceutical applications. He has published more than 200 scientific papers, reviews, and book chapters in internationally renowned journals, as well as edited one book and many journal issues.

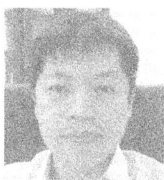

Dr. Jen-Tsung Chen is currently a professor at the National University of Kaohsiung, Taiwan. He teaches cell biology, genomics, proteomics, medicinal plant biotechnology, and plant tissue culture. Dr. Chen's research interests include bioactive compounds, chromatography techniques, *in vitro* culture, medicinal plants, phytochemicals, and plant biotechnology. He has published more than ninety scientific papers and serves as an editorial board member for *Plant Methods*, *Biomolecules*, and *International Journal of Molecular Sciences*.

Contents

Preface

Plants have always been the major source of medicinal bioactive substances. Traditional medicine encompasses the use of plants to cure, diagnose, and prevent disease, as well as to preserve health. As seen by the success of antimalaria artemisinin, traditional medicines are a key source of inspiration for so-called modern medicine, which can contribute to the (re)discovery of new treatments. Artemisinin is not an isolated incidence; several lead bioactive compounds have been discovered in plants used in traditional Chinese, Indian, Japanese, Thai, Korean, African, American, and European medicines. Among these plants, ginseng is the most well-known Chinese medicine and one of the most used herbal medicines, with a wide variety of medicinal and pharmacological applications. *Panax ginseng* C. A. Meyer has been used as a top-grade herb in traditional Chinese medicine or the king of tonic herbs for more than 2,000 years in eastern cultures; the genus name *Panax* means "all-curing" in Greek. Enhancing immunological function, boosting circulation and vascular function, preventing neurological illnesses, modulating metabolism, and promoting vitality and health are only some of the advantages of ginseng preparations. Ginsenosides, commonly known as ginseng saponins or triterpene saponins, are the most important bioactive elements of ginseng. Ginsenosides are exclusively found in ginseng species, and while there are more than 1,000 identified ginsenosides, only a limited number have been tested for biological activity. This book provides an up-to-date critical view of the botanical description and complexity of ginseng, including its phytochemistry, traditional and biotechnological production systems, traditional usage, current applications, and future directions for the development of ginseng compounds as effective medicinal agents. It is a useful resource for academicians, scientists, students, and industry professionals interested in traditional medicine and ginseng.

Dr. Christophe Hano
Department of Biochemistry,
University of Orleans,
Orleans, France

Dr. Jen-Tsung Chen
Department of Life Sciences,
National University of Kaohsiung,
Kaohsiung, Taiwan

Section 1

Introduction

.

Chapter 1

Introductory Chapter: Current Views and Modern Perspectives of Ginseng in Medicines

Christophe Hano and Jen-Tsung Chen

1. Introduction

Ginseng preparations have been widely utilized in many traditional medicines, notably Chinese Traditional Medicine, for approximately 5000 years because of their wide range of medicinal and pharmacological benefits [1]. Ginseng is the generic word for 18 plant species in the Genus *Panax* (Araliaceae), which means "all-curing" in Greek. *Panax ginseng* C. A. Meyer is the most commonly used ginseng in many traditional remedies. Ginseng preparations offer various health benefits, including the promotion of many important physiological functions (e.g., immunity, circulation, and cardiovascular), the prevention of neurological illnesses, the control of energy metabolism, and the maintenance of vitality and health.

The expansion of publications on ginseng, its phytochemistry, and its pharmacological uses over the last 50 years demonstrates that the development of analytical tools and the resurgence of traditional medicine since the 1970s has significantly contributed to rising interest in ginseng (**Figure 1**).

2. Ginseng phytochemistry

The phytochemistry of *Panax* species has been studied since the mid-nineteenth century, with a particular focus on *Panax ginseng* (aka Asian, Chinese, or Korean ginseng)

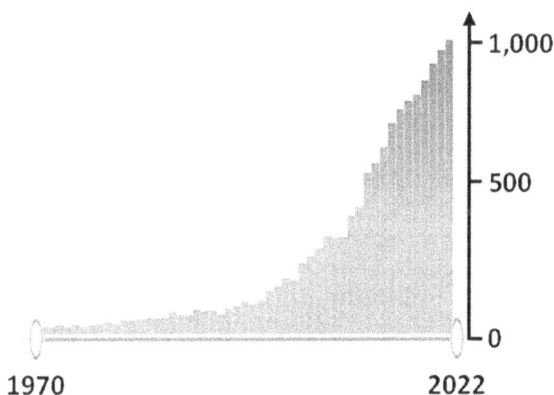

Figure 1.
Publication numbers dealing with ginseng phytochemistry and medicinal uses over the last 50 years (1970–2022).

and *Panax quinquefolius* (aka American ginseng). The most beneficial phytochemicals identified in *Panax* species are ginsenosides (aka ginseng saponins, triterpene saponins). There are around 1000 ginsenosides described to date, Rb1, Rg1, Rg3, Re, Rd., and Rh1 being the most studied ginsenosides. The recent development of new high-throughput analytical instruments and procedures, such as ultra-performance liquid chromatography (UPLC) coupled with high-resolution mass spectrometry (HRMS), has substantially improved our current knowledge of ginsenoside structural diversity [1, 2]. To extract ginsenosides, many extraction processes, including green and modern extraction methods, have been designed, with contents and composition varying widely according to the species, organs, growing season, and production area [3]. Because these approaches allow for the purification of specific ginsenosides, researchers are actively exploiting them to better understand the unique mechanism of ginsenoside activities.

3. Biotechnological approaches

Traditional approaches such as pruning from natural populations or production utilizing a conventional agricultural system can be time-consuming and/or infeasible, paving the way for the development of different biotechnology technologies to improve ginsenoside yield. Thus, various technologies, such as biotechnology, bioconversion, or nanobiotechnology, have been used to overcome these limits. In particular, plant tissue culture has shown to be a useful method for the continuous production of bioactive chemicals [4, 5]. Thus, *in vitro* systems from various plant species, including undifferentiated cell cultures like a callus and cell suspension, as well as differentiated organ cultures like adventitious root and hairy root, have been developed for this purpose over the last decades. For industrial uses, scaling up in bioreactors has also been investigated [4]. The current understanding of ginsenoside biosynthesis and regulation allows for the development of metabolic engineering methods that include not only plant biotechnological systems but also microbial ginsenoside biosynthesis from renewable resources as an alternative strategy for achieving the ever-increasing demand for ginsenosides in recent years [6].

4. Pharmacological development

Antifatigue, antistress, antioxidation, anti-inflammatory, antiaging, anticancer, neuroprotection, and vasorelaxation are only a few of the therapeutic effects of ginseng preparations [1]. The molecular mechanisms and medical applications of ginsenosides have sparked a lot of attention in recent years, with hundreds of studies published (**Figure 1**). Ginsenosides have complex actions and control numerous metabolic pathways, therefore their efficacy is difficult and needs to be further explored. Although various functional studies have been conducted to provide evidence-based research to rationalize traditional usages of ginseng preparations, additional effort is needed to increase therapeutic values using empirical datasets. However, scientists now have a greater opportunity to understand the pharmacological potential of ginseng products and derived ginsenosides, due to the fast development of molecular tools such as high-throughput technologies and integrated multi-omics [7].

Author details

Christophe Hano[1*] and Jen-Tsung Chen[2*]

1 LBLGC, INRAE USC1328, University of Orleans, Chartres, France

2 Department of Life Sciences, National University of Kaohsiung, Kaohsiung, Taiwan

*Address all correspondence to: hano@univ-orleans.fr and jentsung@nuk.edu.tw

IntechOpen

References

[1] Liu L, Xu FR, Wang YZ. Traditional uses, chemical diversity and biological activities of *Panax* L. (Araliaceae): A review. Journal of Ethnopharmacology. 2020;**263**:112792

[2] Yao CL, Pan HQ, Wang H, Yao S, Yang WZ, Hou JJ, et al. Global profiling combined with predicted metabolites screening for discovery of natural compounds: Characterization of ginsenosides in the leaves of *Panax notoginseng* as a case study. Journal of Chromatography A. 2018;**1538**:34-44

[3] Jegal J, Jeong EJ, Yang MH. A review of the different methods applied in ginsenoside extraction from *Panax ginseng* and *Panax quinquefolius* roots. Natural Product Communications. 2019;**14**(9):1934578X19868393

[4] Gantait S, Mitra M, Chen JT. Biotechnological interventions for ginsenosides production. Biomolecules. 2020;**10**(4):538

[5] Liu KH, Lin HY, Thomas JL, Shih YP, Chen JT, Lee MH. Magnetic analogue-imprinted polymers for the extraction of ginsenosides from the *Panax ginseng* callus. Industrial Crops and Products. 2021;**163**:113291

[6] Chu LL, Montecillo JAV, Bae H. Recent advances in the metabolic engineering of yeasts for ginsenoside biosynthesis. Frontiers in Bioengineering and Biotechnology. 2020;**8**:139

[7] Chen JT. Advances in ginsenosides. Biomolecules. 2020;**10**(5):681

Section 2

Phytochemistry and Pharmacology

How Do Extraction Methods and Biotechnology Influence Our Understanding and Usages of Ginsenosides?: A Critical View and Perspectives

Christophe Hano, Duangjai Tungmunnithum, Samantha Drouet, Mohamed Addi, Saikat Gantait and Jen-Tsung Chen

Abstract

Ginseng saponins, *aka* ginsenosides, are bioactive phytochemicals from *Panax* species. *Panax* comes from the Greek word *"panakos,"* which means "cure-all." Owing to their involvement in the creation of numerous medications and nutritional supplements, ginseng saponins play an essential part, especially in the pharmaceutical sector. The main ginsenosides (i.e., Rb1, Rb2, Rc, Rd and Rf) are extracted using a variety of extraction methods, although from a limited number of *Panax* species. However, more than *ca* 1000 unique ginsenosides and 18 *Panax* species have been reported so far, thus demonstrating our present challenge in better understanding of the potential medicinal uses of these compounds. Moreover, ginsenoside production and extraction methods are both time-consuming and inefficient, which has stimulated the development of several efficient extraction and biotechnological technologies to speed up these processes. In this chapter, we highlighted the need to expand the cutting-edge research approaches involving these unique ginsenosides to better understand their biological activities and discover new bioactive ginsenosides as well. The main objective of this chapter is to discuss the undiscovered aspects and limitations of the current biotechnological and extraction technologies, eventually to provide a platform for the production of these unique ginsenosides.

Keywords: biotechnology, extraction methods, ginsenosides, *Panax*, pharmaceutical applications

1. Introduction

The word "ginseng" refers to products that are derived from *Panax* species and relates to the "man-like" form of the root [1]. *Panax ginseng* C. A. Meyer (Araliaceae), sometimes known as Asian, Chinese, or Korean ginseng, and *Panax quinquefolius* L., often known as American or North American ginseng, are the two most well-known ginseng species [2], but a total of 18 plant species, including infraspecific taxa, have been already identified as *Panax* members worldwide [3]. *Panax* is derived from the Greek word "*panakos*," which means "all-healing" or "cure-all," which was first coined by Russian botanist Carl A. Meyer [4]. Thus, the herb ginseng has been used in various traditional medicinal remedies for over 5000 years [4]. Although, different species and parts of ginseng plants have distinct uses in traditional medicine preparations, the root is the most widely used medicinal component of the plant, and saponins are the principal active elements in most of them [5]. Preparations of ginseng dried roots are used to treat hyperglycemia, cardiovascular disease, cancer, and insomnia due to its beneficial biological properties [6–8]. Ginseng is also used as a tonic or adaptogenic supplement that helps to restore biological functions, improve physical performance, and boost tolerance to several stresses [1, 4].

The main bioactive ingredients of *P. ginseng* are a series of tetracyclic triterpenoid saponins also called ginsenosides. In recent years, many excellent reviews on ginsenosides have been published, focusing on structures or bioactivities [1, 8, 9], isolation and analysis [10–13], and metabolic regulation [14–18], thus evidencing our ever-increasing understanding of all these aspects of this thousand-year-old medicinal plant family. However, it is important to keep in mind that the ginsenoside contents greatly vary depending on the species, organs, growing season, and producing location, which implies that their pharmacological properties widely differ as well. Therefore, some important considerations should not be overlooked to continue to improve our understanding:

1. The majority of study relies on the use of Panax extracts, which provide less information regarding their ginsenosides compositions. However, it is important to keep in mind that the phytochemicals accumulated in greater abundance are not necessarily the most active ones.

2. Despite certain similarities, the quantities and the composition of ginsenosides widely differ depending on the *Panax* species, organs, growing season, and producing location. Different ecotypes/natural populations of the same *Panax* species may have substantially different phytochemical profiles.

3. The use of different extraction procedures may generate different types and quantities of ginsenosides (even from the same starting materials). Ginsenosides are categorized based on their polarity, although most studies look at only one kind of solvent, which leads to the production of extracts with very similar ginsenoside compositions. As a result, our ability to discover novel bioactive ginsenosides and/or biological activity is severely limited.

4. Traditional plant propagation takes around six years and is inconvenient for proper industrial production, which in turn has led to the involvement of biotechnological approaches, notably *in vitro* culture, to provide fast and continuous access to bioactive *Panax* extracts. However, the phytochemical profiles of these *in vitro* cultures, might significantly differ, both in terms of ginsenoside quantities and compositions, from those of the initial explants.

Although, all of these differences in ginsenoside contents and compositions may appear to be disadvantageous or anecdotal, we have decided to highlight them in this chapter to emphasize that they may, on the contrary, be an asset to our understanding of ginsenoside biological activity and discovery of new bioactive ginsenosides.

2. A Tour d'Horizon of the Ginsenosides chemical diversity

Initially, the term "ginsenosides" was used to design a series of tetracyclic triterpenoid saponins from *P. ginseng*. According to different aglycones, triterpenoid saponins may be classified into tetracyclic triterpene saponins (e.g., dammarane-type saponins, DAMS) and pentacyclic triterpene saponins (e.g., oleanolic-type (OT) and ocotillol-type (OA) saponins). The main aglycones of which are protopanaxadiol (PPD), protopanaxatriol (PPT), oleanolic acid, and ocotillol [1, 11]. A variety of saponins are biosynthesized with different types of glycosides groups and/or linkage orders. DAMS, such as PPTs and PPDs, generally contain 1 to 4 glycosyl groups linked with the aglycone structure. Sugar chains are usually linked to the C3 or C4 position of the aglycone in PPD type saponins, whereas regularly linked to the C6 or C20 position in PPT type saponins.

The ginsenoside chemical annotation is 'Rx', where 'R' stands for root and 'x' stands for chromatographic polarity in alphabetical order. To date, the Rb (protopanaxadiols) and the Rg groups (protopanaxatriols) are the most studied ones (**Figure 1**). With the availability of commercial standards, these ginsenosides Rb1, Rb2, Rc, and Rd from the Rb group (or PPD), and the ginsenosides Rg1, Rg2, Re, and Rf from the Rg group (or PPT) (**Figure 1**) were more readily analyzed during the extraction procedure, thus leading in greater available information on their biological activity.

Panax plant phytochemistry has been investigated since the mid-nineteenth century, mostly with *P. ginseng* or *P. quinquefolius* as starting materials. Samuel S. Garrigues isolated the first ginsenoside, "panaquilon," from *P. quinquefolius* roots in 1854 [19]. Due to the renewed interest in natural compounds and traditional medicines, various unique *Panax* species, such as *P. vietnamensis* Ha et Grushv. and *P. sokpayensis*, have piqued the interest of many phytochemists since 1970s [20, 21]. Between 1970 and 2000, owing to the development and democratization in laboratory techniques such as two-dimensional nuclear magnetic resonance (2D NMR) or quadrupole time of flight mass spectrometry (Q-TOF-MS) that were employed to detect *Panax* chemical components and clarify stereo configurations, it was found that the structures of many saponin compounds mostly belonged to C17 side-chain that varied for both PPD- and PPT-type ginsenosides [22–26]. But since the 2000s, an impressive and growing number of new saponins have been

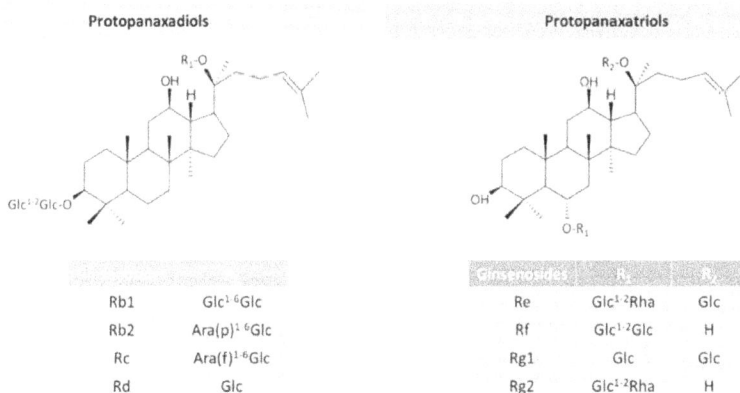

Protopanaxadiols				Protopanaxatriols		
	Rb1	Glc$^{1-6}$Glc		Ginsenosides	R$_1$	R$_2$
	Rb2	Ara(p)$^{1-6}$Glc		Re	Glc$^{1-2}$Rha	Glc
	Rc	Ara(f)$^{1-6}$Glc		Rf	Glc$^{1-2}$Glc	H
	Rd	Glc		Rg1	Glc	Glc
				Rg2	Glc$^{1-2}$Rha	H

Figure 1.
Chemical structure of Panax species' common protopanaxadiol (PPD or Rb) and protopanaxatriol (PPT or Rg) ginsenosides.

discovered owing to the significant advances in chromatography, spectroscopy and mass spectrometry methods that allow rapid and efficient screening of natural *Panax* products. The work of Yao et al. [27] perfectly illustrated this impressive progress by resolving 945 ginsenosides from the leaves of *P. notoginseng* by using two-dimensional liquid chromatography (2D-LC) separation technology, based on high-performance liquid chromatography coupled with high-resolution mass spectrometry (HPLC-HRMS) platform, 662 of which were novel.

From this brief historical background, it is indisputable that the emergence of more efficient analytical approaches has substantially improved our understanding of the chemical variety of ginsenosides. Here are some additional important observations on the chemical diversity to be taken into account for future development (beginning with the most well-known compounds):

1. There are 94 PPD-type ginsenosides known to date. Their sugar moieties are linked to the C3 and/or C20 position(s) (e.g., Rb1, Rb2, Rc, and Rd, **Figure 1**), while acylation, particularly of the 6-OH function of the C3 glucose, has been reported. It is now undeniable that acylation is a key source of new structures in PPDs, and it deserves more attention both from chemical and biological perspectives.

2. There are 93 PPT-type ginsenosides described. Typically, the sugar moieties are linked to the ring at the C6 position (e.g., Rg1, Re, and Rg5, **Figure 1**), and possibly at the C20 position. In addition, some other interesting substitutions have been reported as well. For instance, the direct substitution of malonyl or acetyl at the C-6′ or C-3 positions appeared to boost antiproliferative activity [1], or the presence of an olefine acid ester group and acetyl at the C-6 position has been linked to significant inhibition of antimycin A-induced mitochondrial oxidative stress [28]. These two examples highlight the necessity of focusing on new structures and extended structure-function studies to increase our current understanding of PPT ginsenosides' pharmaceutical potential.

3. The 34 OA- and 23 OT-type ginsenosides forms a minor group of ginsenosides. The main OA-type ginsenoside Ro is thought to be biosynthesized from oleanolic acid, and was initially identified in trace amounts in *P. ginseng*. OT-type ginsenosides are tetracyclic triterpene saponins with a furan ring on the side chain as described in *P. pseudoginseng*, *P. quinquefolius*, *P. vietnamensis* and *P. japonicus* extracts. Further research on these chemicals is required to characterize their medicinal potentials. In addition, the chemotaxonomic and authentication potentials of these OA and OT compounds should be further explored.

4. Around 220 saponins with C-17 varied side chain (including lupane-triterpenes) and 53 others structural saponins (465–516) have been reported to date. Some lupane-triterpene compounds have demonstrated effective anti-inflammatory activity acting on various targets (inhibition of cyclooxygenase-2 (COX2), decrease in cellular NO synthase (iNOS) concentrations) [29]. This also emphasizes the importance of exploring even the "minor" (in accumulation concentrations) ginsenoside structures for future pharmaceutical product development.

3. A critical evaluation of the analytical procedures used in the extraction of ginsenosides

Over the last decades, different extraction procedures were studied and have yielded different kinds and quantities of ginsenosides. A recent review has comprehensively compilated the different results obtained [11]. So far, the bulk of studies to far have focused on two Panax species (*P. ginseng* and *P. quinquefolius*) and a small number of ginsenosides (mainly the Rb and Rg type ginsenosides). Here, we combined the various processes utilized to extract these main ginsenosides from the roots of *P. ginseng* and *P. quinquefolius* so that we could compare the results and draw conclusions as well as future directions (**Table 1**).

This review of the literature found a wide range of variations in the ginsenoside extraction yields [from 1.0 [51] to 79.5 mg/g DW [36]], with no extraction approach appearing to be ideal. However, given our previous observations on the variability of these ginsenoside contents (which varied greatly depending on the species, organs, growing season, and production location), and the fact that the majority of these studies did not use different types of starting material to eliminate these variabilities associated with this material, it is difficult to draw firm conclusions from these data. Nevertheless, based on the critical analysis of **Table 1**, the following critical observations can be made:

1. Traditional extraction methods such as Soxhlet and heat reflux (**Figure 2**) yielded a wide range of ginsenoside content in *P. ginseng* and *P. quinquefolius*, depending on the solvent, extraction time, and sample preparation. High ginsenoside content can be achieved, but at the expense of a long extraction time and/or a high temperature, both of which are costly in terms of energy use.

2. The use of modern extraction methods (ultrasound, microwave, high pressure) (**Figure 2**) can be a good alternative to these traditional extraction procedures, since they are less time-consuming, need less solvent, are readily automated, and result in higher extraction yields. Extraction using high pressure or pressurized liquid (e.g., accelerated solvent extraction or pressurized fluid extraction) dramatically enhanced extraction yields and considerably reduced extraction time.

3. There were no consistent direct proportional connections found between ginsenoside extraction yield and extraction parameters (solvent concentration, extraction pressure, and extraction time).

4. However, it appeared that the ginsenoside extraction yield can be greatly influenced by solvent use. However, it was notable that only a restricted number of solvents with very similar polarity were evaluated. Given the vast range of variations that were observed for the various ginsenosides (especially for the less studied ones), more solvents should be investigated in the future. Natural deep eutectic solvents, for instance, may have a greater range of extraction capability and might be a good option to investigate a wider range of ginsenosides, as recently demonstrated by Liu et al. [53].

5. In this context, supercritical carbon dioxide extraction (**Figure 2**) emerged as an appealing approach for studying less polar ginsenosides. However, for compounds with higher polarity, the polarity of the fluid phase must be

Species [1]		Solvent	Duration (min)	Other parameters	Ginsenosides				References
Pg	Pq				Rb	Rg	Others	TOTAL	
Soxhlet									
■		Water/n-BuOH	480					24.6	[30]
	■	Water/n-BuOH	480					46.1	[30]
■		70% EtOH	300	60°C, 0.1 Mpa				22.2	[31]
■		70% EtOH	360	75°C				29.6	[32]
■		70% EtOH	360	90°C				42.8	[33]
	■	95% EtOH	480	70°C					[34]
■		100% MeOH	60					23.8	[35]
	■	100% MeOH	60					79.5	[36]
■		100% MeOH	20	140°C, 3Mpa				17.2	[37]
	■	100% MeOH	20	140°C, 3Mpa				38.8	[37]
	■	100% MeOH	1200					75.5	[38]
Heat Reflux									
■		Water	60	95°C				1.3 *	[39]
	■	Water	90	100°C					[40]
■		50% EtOH	240					57.5	[41]
	■	50% EtOH	360	70°C					[42]
■		70% EtOH	360	80°C				18.6	[41]
■		70% EtOH	360	80°C				7.2	[42]
■		70% EtOH	240	80°C				43.3	[33]
■		80% MeOH	180	75°C				36.2	[43]
	■	100% MeOH	60	60°C				52.1	[44]
Shaking									
■		Water	1440	25°C, 0.1Mpa				9.2	[45]
	■	50% MeOH	60					41.0	[46]
Ultasound									
■		Water/n-BuOH	120	25°C				24.5	[30]
	■	Water/n-BuOH	120					7.2	[47]
■		50% EtOH	30					58.9	[41]
■		70% EtOH	60	25°C				6.8	[42]
■		70% EtOH	40	60°C				38.9	[33]
	■	70% EtOH	40						[34]
■		70% EtOH	240	70°C				14.5	[41]
■		70% EtOH	180	70°C				31.1	[32]
	■	50% MeOH	60					26.1	[46]

							Total	
Microwave								
	70% EtOH	10					9.8	[41]
	70% EtOH	10					7.2	[42]
	70% EtOH	10					33.0	[33]
	70% EtOH	15						[48]
	70% EtOH	15	0.5Mpa				36.4	[31]
	70% EtOH	15						[34]
Pressurized Liquid								
	Water	30	110°C, 0.4Mpa				11.2	[47]
	70% EtOH	5	150°C, 6.7Mpa				8.7	[42]
	50% MeOH	25	120°C, 10Mpa				26.0	[46]
	100% MeOH	15	150°C, 10.3Mpa				58.9	[49]
	100% MeOH	15	150°C, 6.9Mpa				62.2	[50]
	100% MeOH	15	150°C, 6.9Mpa				18.6	[50]
	100% MeOH	20	140°C, 3Mpa				12.9	[37]
	100% MeOH	20	140°C, 3Mpa				39.2	[37]
Supercritical Fluid								
	100% CO$_2$	240					1.0	[51]
	100% CO$_2$	240	45°C, 24Mpa				23.2	[41]
	100% CO$_2$	240	40°C, 30Mpa				3.2	[34]
	100% CO$_2$	1200	110°C, 48.3Mpa				71.8	[38]
High-Pressure/Microwave								
	70% EtOH	10	0.4Mpa				43.3	[36]
	70% EtOH	11	0.5Mpa				49.4	[52]
Ultrahigh-Pressure								
	Water	5	25°C, 300Mpa				23.8	[45]
	50% EtOH	2	500Mpa				73.3	[41]
	50% EtOH	2	25°C, 200Mpa					[34]
	70% EtOH	5	25°C, 200Mpa				11.9	[43]
	70% EtOH	5	60°C, 200Mpa				43.9	[33]

[1]P. ginseng *and* P. quinquefolius.
The relative concentrations of the widely investigated Rb and Rg ginsenosides were shown by the colors (blue = low,
red – high, orange – detected but not quantified), and the resulting total ginsenosides content was given in the column "Total."

Table 1.
Variations in ginsenoside content were obtained using different extraction procedures from the two most frequently investigated Panax species [30–53].

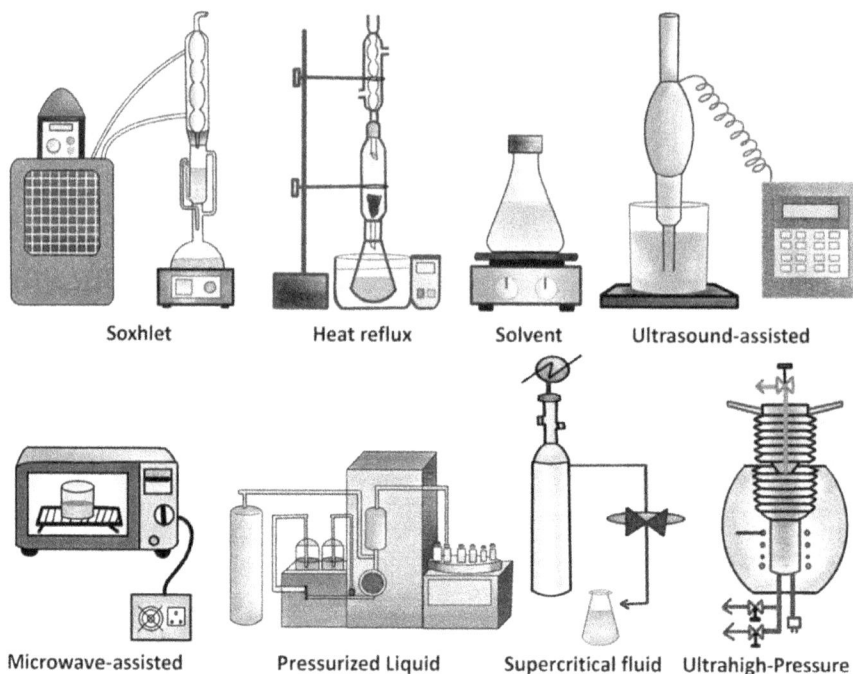

Figure 2.
Diagrams showing different traditional and modern methods used for ginsenoside extraction.

increased during extraction with supercritical carbon dioxide and a small addition of polar modifiers like methanol, ethanol or DMSO.

6. In the future, more *Panax* species and ginsenoside structures should be investigated, particularly utilizing modern tools and techniques. In this context, for those ginsenosides that accumulated in lower concentrations, cutting-edge techniques such as macroporous resins or, more interestingly, magnetic analogue-imprinted polymers with high capacity and selectivity have been highlighted [54], should be considered.

4. A critical look at biotechnological interventions to ginsenoside bioproduction

The conventional approaches for ginsenoside pruning from natural populations or production using the classical agricultural systems can be time-consuming and/or not feasible, and thus it has paved the way for the development of various biotechnological approaches, which would ameliorate the productivity of ginsenosides. Plant tissue culture proved to be an important tool for the continuous production of bioactive compounds that are specialized metabolites in most of the instances. However, the notion of productivity is essential here, and it is far more significant than production. Naturally, secondary metabolites (*aka* specialized metabolites) are produced from primary metabolites (such as carbohydrates, lipids, and amino acids) that are required for plant growth and development. The key concern is that if the primary metabolites are involved too actively for the biosynthesis of a specific class of specialized metabolite, plant growth and development may deteriorate eventually. As a result, high productivity collectively defined as *"biomass x production yield of bioactive specialized metabolite"* is significantly more desirable for efficient and continuous output of specialized metabolite at the industrial level.

For this purpose, *in vitro* systems (**Figure 3a**) for various plant species have been developed over the last decades, including undifferentiated cell cultures like a callus and cell suspension, as well as differentiated organ cultures like adventitious root and hairy root, with widely disparate results in terms of biomass production and/or ginsenoside accumulation, as recently reviewed by Gantait et al. [18].

The most notable results of these various plant biotechnology techniques are critically reviewed below, along with some perspectives:

1. During a critical evaluation of the analytical procedures developed for the extraction of ginsenosides, we observed that only a limited number of *Panax* species, as well as a small number of different ginsenosides, have been thoroughly investigated with the aid of biotechnological methods to date.

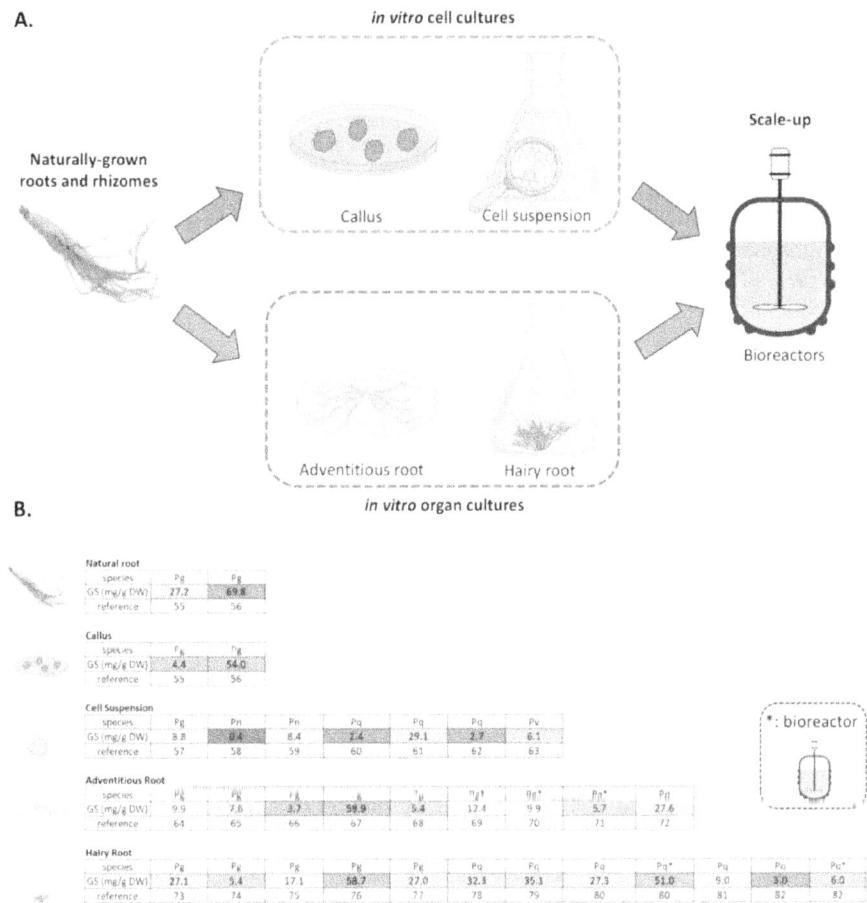

Figure 3.
*a. Flowchart depicting the main biotechnology approaches that have been developed using the various plant in vitro culture systems; b. Comparison of the total ginsenoside production (GS) obtained using various plant in vitro culture systems (callus, cell suspension, adventitious root and hairy root compared to naturally grown rhizome). * production done in a bioreactor; DW: dry weight. Pg: P. ginseng; Pq: P. quinquefolius; Pn: P. notoginseng; Pv: P. vietnamensis [55–82].*

2. The total ginsenoside contents greatly varied from more than 2 orders of magnitude (from 0.4 mg/g DW in *P. notoginseng* cell suspension culture [58] to 59.9 mg/g DW for *P. ginseng* adventitious root culture [67] as a function of the considered *Panax* species, but also the type of in vitro system and growing conditions (**Figure 3b**).

3. When comparing *in vitro* cell cultures (callus and/or cell suspension) to naturally-cultivated ginseng root, it can be shown that *in vitro* cultures (callus and/or cell suspension) yielded 6-times less ginsenosides [55]. However, *in vitro* cell cultures can product massive and continuous biomass. Cell suspensions are more promising option than callus cultures for this purpose owing to their possibility to be scaled-up in a bioreactor. In addition, cell suspensions are obtained from a single cell or a small number of more genetically homogenous cells, hence they are commonly more stable in terms of growth and metabolite production capacities than callus cultures. On the other hand, callus cultures are usually a chimera of cells with very contrasting genetic profiles, resulting in contrasting and unstable growth and/or production profiles. For all of these reasons, cell suspensions are preferred for production, although calli are subjects of interest from a fundamental viewpoint to explore a wide range of developmental phases and thereby uncovering unusual ginsenoside accumulation profiles, both quantitatively and qualitatively.

4. Differentiated *in vitro* root-derived cultures, particularly in the case of hairy root, are promising *in vitro* production systems both in terms of biomass and ginsenoside production yields. This might be because ginsenoside is produced naturally in the root and rhizome. Furthermore, both adventitious and hairy roots may be scaled up in a bioreactor [69–71, 80, 82].

5. The selection of fast-growing and high-producing lines is an essential preliminary step before considering large-scale stable production since these parameters are highly variable [75]. Screening a large number of both wild-type [56, 75] or mutant [77] lines verified this interest. It has been demonstrated to contribute in the identification of certain lines capable of producing a single ginsenoside at significant levels [75]. It should be underlined that starting from different genotypes, cultivars or populations for the initiation of *in vitro* cultures may be especially significant for this purpose and have been largely unexplored.

6. The composition of plant culture medium is a significant factor in both the growth and the production of specialized metabolites. Therefore, the cultural conditions must be adjusted. For example, the production of various ginsenosides has been demonstrated to be dependent on the growing culture phase, as evidenced by several PPD derivatives [59, 78]. This is especially true for bioreactor production for which oxygenation is essential [71].

7. Elicitation strategies can have a significant impact on total ginsenoside yields. In particular, jasmonates (jasmonate, methyl-jasmonate, and 2-hydroxyethyl-jasmonate) have been extensively studied and found to enhance total ginsenoside production [57, 58, 76, 77, 80]. But, more interestingly, various jasmonate derivatives have been shown to preferentially stimulate PPD-type ginsenosides over PPT-type ginsenosides, indicating that it might be an

appealing option for redirecting ginsenoside biosynthesis [77]. It should be emphasized that elicitation has usually resulted in a reduction in growth [76].

8. Too infrequently, detailed metabolic investigation of the ginsenoside accumulation patterns has been investigated. The majority of investigations focused on total ginsenoside content or a limited number of ginsenosides. The study by Ha et al. [83] on the hairy roots of *P. vietnamensis* nicely demonstrated the benefits of in-depth LC-MS characterization for the discovery of unique accumulation patterns.

The current understanding of ginsenoside biosynthesis and regulation paves the way for metabolic engineering strategies to be developed [17]. For this purpose, in addition to the plant *in vitro* cultures, the microbial biosynthesis of ginsenosides from renewable resources may be a viable alternative technique for meeting the ever-increasing demand for ginsenosides in recent years [16]. Microbes have several benefits over plant cells, including the need for less area for growth, the ability to grow quickly with high cell density culture, the ability to regulate and describe genetics, and the ability to manipulate genetics. Yeasts, particularly *Saccharomyces cerevisiae*, are well-known as eukaryotic model organisms for the creation of high-value compounds with complex structures. In recent years, alternative approaches for ginsenoside production have been developed using the model yeast *Saccharomyces cerevisiae* and non-conventional yeasts such as *Yarrowia lipolytica* and *Pichia pastoris* [16].

5. Conclusions

"What you see is what you extract" remarked Y.H. Choi and R. Verpootre [84]. This is especially true for ginsenosides. Most extraction methods continue to focus only on the major bioactive ginsenosides, although more holistic approaches to extraction-based research would substantially increase our understanding of the biological activities of this family of natural products. As critically discussed in the present chapter, ginsenosides may not have provided their full potential as medicinal resources due to a global lack of effective technologies for ginsenoside extraction and/or production.

The majority of the extraction procedures involve the most common bioactive components only (i.e., PPD-type ginsenosides: Rg3, Rb1, Rb2, Rc, and Rd; and PPT-type ginsenosides: Rg1, Re, and Rg5) from a limited number of *Panax* species (*P. ginseng* and *P. quinquefolius* mainly). On the contrary, some species, like *P. sokpayensis* and *P. stipuleanatus*, have received little attention. Additional bioactive components may be found using bioactivity-oriented separation methods. Further research will be needed to understand the molecular and cellular processes, toxicity using cellular and animal models, and clinical applications of less-studied ginsenosides. This would allow for more in-depth research of the structure-activity relationships of ginsenosides, which would provide important insights into the development of a *Panax* quality control method, based on faster and more accurate analytical procedures. In addition, the development of more effective holistic strategies vis-a-vis more specific targeted extraction procedures would go a long way toward ensuring that the *Panax* species continues to reveal new secrets. It is feasible to generate richer extracts through a more precise extraction strategy (for example, using NaDES combined with ultrasonic or high-pressure extraction) and then fractionate this extract with much more specific extraction methods for certain classes of ginsenosides (e.g., with bio-imprinted polymers).

Biotechnological production of different ginsenosides using *in vitro* cultures has not been thoroughly investigated to date, nor have quantitative analyses of less common ginsenosides been undertaken. Although, there have been several publications on cell suspension cultures and bioreactors, the use of elicitors has to be investigated more often, using omics technologies (metabolomics and transcriptomics) to provide full insight, since these compounds may have a substantial influence on ginsenoside biosynthesis. Recently, the microbial cell factory has been proposed as a source of the production of main ginsenosides, for which biosynthetic genes have been isolated. In this sense, plant and microbial biotechnology approaches are complementary: plant can reveal new structures, in particular, using elicitation coupled to omics studies and allow the identification of new genes that can then be used in both plant metabolic engineering or microbial synthetic biology approaches.

Panax species have been widely employed in traditional medicine and are known to have pharmaceutical uses. Ginsenosides have only recently been studied, owing to advances in analytical methods since the first comprehensive phytochemical descriptions in the 1970s. The current surge in the application of advanced technologies, such as HR-MS, has enabled the discovery of an increasing number of ginsenoside structures. These unique structures have not yet been explored due to their most recent discovery, and a lack of availability of adequate quantity.

Acknowledgements

C.H. and D.T. gratefully acknowledge the support of Campus France and the French Embassy in Thailand through the PHC SIAM (PNPIA, Project 44926WK). D.T. and C.H. acknowledge Le Studium Institute for Advance Study for its support. D.T. is thankful to Mahidol University. C.H. and S.D. acknowledge the support of Département d'Eure et Loir (Eure & Loir Campus), ARD CosmétoSciences (Loire Valley Region) and ARD Biomédicaments (Loire Valley Region). S.D. acknowledges research fellowship of Loire Valley Region.

Conflict of interest

The authors declare no conflict of interest.

Author details

Christophe Hano[1*], Duangjai Tungmunnithum[2], Samantha Drouet[1], Mohamed Addi[3], Saikat Gantait[4] and Jen-Tsung Chen[5]

1 LBLGC, INRAE USC1328, University of Orleans, Chartres, France

2 Faculty of Pharmacy, Department of Pharmaceutical Botany, Mahidol University, Bangkok, Thailand

3 Laboratoire d'Amélioration des Productions Agricoles, Biotechnologie et Environnement (LAPABE), Faculté des Sciences, Université Mohammed Premier, Oujda, Morocco

4 Crop Research Unit (Genetics and Plant Breeding), Bidhan Chandra Krishi Viswavidyalaya, Nadia, West Bengal, India

5 Department of Life Sciences, National University of Kaohsiung, Kaohsiung, Taiwan

*Address all correspondence to: hano@univ-orleans.fr

IntechOpen

References

[1] Liu L, Xu FR, Wang YZ. Traditional uses, chemical diversity and biological activities of *Panax* L. (Araliaceae): A review. Journal of Ethnopharmacology. 2020;**263**:112792

[2] Jia L, Zhao Y. Current evaluation of the millennium phytomedicine-ginseng (I): Etymology, pharmacognosy, phytochemistry, market and regulations. Current Medicinal Chemistry. 2009;**16**(19):2475-2484

[3] Yahara S, Tanaka O, Nishioka I. Dammarane Type Saponins of Leaves of Panax japonicus CA MEYER. (2).: Saponins of the Specimens collected in Tottori-ken, Kyoto-shi, and Niigata-ken. Chemical and Pharmaceutical Bulletin. 1978;**26**(10):3010-3016

[4] Baranov A. Recent advances in our knowledge of the morphology, cultivation and uses of ginseng (*Panax ginseng* CA Meyer). Economic Botany. 1966;**20**(4):403-406

[5] Bai M, Mao Q, Xu JD, Zhu LY, Zhu H, Wang Q, et al. Advance in saponins of aerial parts of *Panax* species. *Zhongguo Zhong yao za zhi= Zhongguo zhongyao zazhi=*. China Journal of Chinese Materia Medica. 2014;**39**(3):412-422

[6] Yin J, Zhang H, Ye J. Traditional Chinese medicine in treatment of metabolic syndrome. Endocrine, Metabolic & Immune Disorders-Drug Targets (Formerly Current Drug Targets-Immune Endocrine & Metabolic Disorders). 2008;**8**(2):99-111

[7] Zhou W, Chai H, Lin PH, Lumsden AB, Yao Q, Chen C. Molecular mechanisms and clinical applications of ginseng root for cardiovascular disease. Medical Science Monitor. 2004;**10**(8): RA187-RA192

[8] Shin BK, Kwon SW, Park JH. Chemical diversity of ginseng saponins from *Panax ginseng*. Journal of Ginseng Research. 2015;**39**(4):287-298

[9] Wang T, Guo R, Zhou G, Zhou X, Kou Z, Sui F, et al. Traditional uses, botany, phytochemistry, pharmacology and toxicology of *Panax notoginseng* (Burk.) FH Chen: A review. Journal of Ethnopharmacology. 2016;**188**:234-258

[10] Wang Y, Choi HK, Brinckmann JA, Jiang X, Huang L. Chemical analysis of *Panax quinquefolius* (North American ginseng): A review. Journal of Chromatography A. 2015;**1426**:1-15

[11] Jegal J, Jeong EJ, Yang MH. A review of the different methods applied in ginsenoside extraction from *Panax ginseng* and *Panax quinquefolius* roots. Natural Product Communications. 2019; **14**(9):1934578X19868393

[12] Xu C, Wang W, Wang B, Zhang T, Cui X, Pu Y, et al. Analytical methods and biological activities of *Panax notoginseng* saponins: Recent trends. Journal of Ethnopharmacology. 2019; **236**:443-465

[13] Yang Y, Ju Z, Yang Y, Zhang Y, Yang L, Wang Z. Phytochemical analysis of *Panax* species: A review. Journal of Ginseng Research. 2021;**45**(1): 1-21

[14] Paek KY, Murthy HN, Hahn EJ, Zhong JJ. Large scale culture of ginseng adventitious roots for production of ginsenosides. Biotechnology in China. 2009;**I**:151-176

[15] Rahimi S, Kim YJ, Yang DC. Production of ginseng saponins: Elicitation strategy and signal transductions. Applied Microbiology and Biotechnology. 2015;**99**(17):6987-6996

[16] Chu LL, Montecillo JAV, Bae H. Recent advances in the metabolic

engineering of yeasts for ginsenoside biosynthesis. Frontiers in Bioengineering and Biotechnology. 2020;**8**:139

[17] Hou M, Wang R, Zhao S, Wang Z. Ginsenosides in *Panax* genus and their biosynthesis. Acta Pharmaceutica Sinica B. 2021;**11**(7):1813-1834

[18] Gantait S, Mitra M, Chen JT. Biotechnological interventions for ginsenosides production. Biomolecules. 2020;**10**(4):538

[19] Garrigues SS. Chemical Investigations on Radix Ginseng Americana, Oleum Chenopodii Anthelmintici and Oleum Menthae Viridis. Göttingen: Univ, Diss, EA Huth; 1854

[20] Yamasaki K, Tanaka O. Saponins from Vietnamese ginseng, *Panax vietnamensis* HA et Grushv. Collected in central Vietnam. II. Chemical and Pharmaceutical Bulletin. 1994;**42**(1): 115-122

[21] Sharma SK, Pandit MK. A new species of *Panax* L. (Araliaceae) from Sikkim Himalaya, India. Systematic Botany. 2009;**34**(2):434-438

[22] Ma WG, Mizutani M, Malterud KE, Lu SL, Ducrey B, Tahara S. Saponins from the roots of *Panax notoginseng*. Phytochemistry. 1999;**52**(6):1133-1139

[23] Wang HP, Zhang YB, Yang XW, Zhao DQ, Wang YP. Rapid characterization of ginsenosides in the roots and rhizomes of *Panax ginseng* by UPLC-DAD-QTOF-MS/MS and simultaneous determination of 19 ginsenosides by HPLC-ESI-MS. Journal of Ginseng Research. 2016;**40**(4): 382-394

[24] Wang MM, Xue M, Xu YG, Miao Y, Kou N, Yang L, et al. *Panax notoginseng* saponin is superior to aspirin in inhibiting platelet adhesion to injured endothelial cells through COX pathway *in vitro*. Thrombosis Research. 2016;**141**: 146-152

[25] Wang P, Du X, Xiong M, Cui J, Yang Q, Wang W, et al. Ginsenoside Rd attenuates breast cancer metastasis implicating derepressing microRNA-18a-regulated Smad2 expression. Scientific Reports. 2016;**6**(1):1-14

[26] Wang Y, Ren Y, Xing L, Dai X, Liu S, Yu B, et al. Endothelium-dependent vasodilation effects of *Panax notoginseng* and its main components are mediated by nitric oxide and cyclooxygenase pathways. Experimental and Therapeutic Medicine. 2016;**12**(6): 3998-4006

[27] Yao CL, Pan HQ, Wang H, Yao S, Yang WZ, Hou JJ, et al. Global profiling combined with predicted metabolites screening for discovery of natural compounds: Characterization of ginsenosides in the leaves of *Panax notoginseng* as a case study. Journal of Chromatography A. 2018;**1538**:34-44

[28] Zhang Y, Han LF, Sakah KJ, Wu ZZ, Liu LL, Agyemang K, et al. Bioactive protopanaxatriol type saponins isolated from the roots of *Panax notoginseng* (Burk.) FH Chen. Molecules. 2013; **18**(9):10352-10366

[29] Kim JA, Son JH, Yang SY, Song SB, Song GY, Kim YH. A new lupane-type triterpene from the seeds of Panax ginseng with its inhibition of NF-κB. Archives of Pharmacal Research. 2012; **35**(4):647-651

[30] Wu J, Lin L, Chau FT. Ultrasound-assisted extraction of ginseng saponins from ginseng roots and cultured ginseng cells. Ultrasonics Sonochemistry. 2001; **8**(4):347-352

[31] Shi W, Wang Y, Li J, Zhang H, Ding L. Investigation of ginsenosides in different parts and ages of *Panax*

ginseng. Food Chemistry. 2007;**102**(3): 664-668

[32] Hu JN, Lee JH, Shin JA, Choi JE, Lee KT. Determination of ginsenosides content in Korean ginseng seeds and roots by high performance liquid chromatography. Food Science and Biotechnology. 2008;**17**(2):430-433

[33] Chen R, Meng F, Zhang S, Liu Z. Effects of ultrahigh pressure extraction conditions on yields and antioxidant activity of ginsenoside from ginseng. Separation and Purification Technology. 2009;**66**(2):340-346

[34] Zhang S, Chen R, Wu H, Wang C. Ginsenoside extraction from *Panax quinquefolium* L. (American ginseng) root by using ultrahigh pressure. Journal of Pharmaceutical and Biomedical Analysis. 2006;**41**(1):57-63

[35] Wang CZ, Aung HH, Ni M, Wu JA, Tong R, Wicks S, et al. Red American ginseng: Ginsenoside constituents and antiproliferative activities of heat-processed *Panax quinquefolius* roots. Planta Medica. 2007;**73**(07):669-674

[36] Wang Y, You J, Yu Y, Qu C, Zhang H, Ding L, et al. Analysis of ginsenosides in *Panax ginseng* in high pressure microwave-assisted extraction. Food Chemistry. 2008;**110**(1):161-167

[37] Wang X, Sakuma T, Asafu-Adjaye E, Shiu GK. Determination of ginsenosides in plant extracts from *Panax ginseng* and *Panax quinquefolius* L. by LC/MS/MS. Analytical Chemistry. 1999;**71**(8):1579-1584

[38] Wood JA, Bernards MA, Wan WK, Charpentier PA. Extraction of ginsenosides from North American ginseng using modified supercritical carbon dioxide. The Journal of Supercritical Fluids. 2006;**39**(1):40-47

[39] Lee HS, Lee HJ, Yu HJ, Ju DW, Kim Y, Kim CT, et al. A comparison between high hydrostatic pressure extraction and heat extraction of ginsenosides from ginseng (*Panax ginseng* CA Meyer). Journal of the Science of Food and Agriculture. 2011;**91**(8):1466-1473

[40] Popovich DG, Kitts DD. Generation of ginsenosides Rg3 and Rh2 from North American ginseng. Phytochemistry. 2004;**65**(3):337-344

[41] Shouqin Z, Ruizhan C, Changzheng W. Experiment study on ultrahigh pressure extraction of ginsenosides. Journal of Food Engineering. 2007; **79**(1):1-5

[42] Hou J, He S, Ling M, Li W, Dong R, Pan Y, et al. A method of extracting ginsenosides from *Panax ginseng* by pulsed electric field. Journal of Separation Science. 2010;**33**(17–18): 2707-2713

[43] Kwon JH, Belanger JM, Pare JJ, Yaylayan VA. Application of the microwave-assisted process (MAP™) to the fast extraction of ginseng saponins. Food Research International. 2003;**36**(5): 491-498

[44] Corbit RM, Ferreira JF, Ebbs SD, Murphy LL. Simplified extraction of ginsenosides from American ginseng (*Panax quinquefolius* L.) for high-performance liquid chromatography–ultraviolet analysis. Journal of Agricultural and Food Chemistry. 2005; **53**(26):9867-9873

[45] Shin JS, Ahn SC, Choi SW, Lee DU, Kim BY, Baik MY. Ultra-high-pressure extraction (UHPE) of ginsenosides from Korean *Panax ginseng* powder. Food Science and Biotechnology. 2010;**19**(3): 743-748

[46] Ligor T, Ludwiczuk A, Wolski T, Buszewski B. Isolation and determination of ginsenosides in American ginseng leaves and root extracts by LC-MS. Analytical and

Bioanalytical Chemistry. 2005;**383**(7): 1098-1105

[47] Engelberth AS, Clausen EC, Carrier DJ. Comparing extraction methods to recover ginseng saponins from American ginseng (*Panax quinquefolium*), followed by purification using fast centrifugal partition chromatography with HPLC verification. Separation and Purification Technology. 2010;**72**(1):1-6

[48] Shu YY, Ko MY, Chang YS. Microwave-assisted extraction of ginsenosides from ginseng root. Microchemical Journal. 2003;**74**(2): 131-139

[49] Qian ZM, Lu J, Gao QP, Li SP. Rapid method for simultaneous determination of flavonoid, saponins and polyacetylenes in Folium Ginseng and Radix Ginseng by pressurized liquid extraction and high-performance liquid chromatography coupled with diode array detection and mass spectrometry. Journal of Chromatography A. 2009; **1216**(18):3825-3830

[50] Wan JB, Li SP, Chen JM, Wang YT. Chemical characteristics of three medicinal plants of the *Panax* genus determined by HPLC-ELSD. Journal of Separation Science. 2007;**30**(6):825-832

[51] Luo D, Qiu T, Lu Q. Ultrasound-assisted extraction of ginsenosides in supercritical CO_2 reverse microemulsions. Journal of the Science of Food and Agriculture. 2007;**87**(3): 431-436

[52] Qu C, Bai Y, Jin X, Wang Y, Zhang K, You J, et al. Study on ginsenosides in different parts and ages of *Panax quinquefolius* L. Food Chemistry. 2009; **115**(1):340-346

[53] Liu X, Ahlgren S, Korthout HA, Salomé-Abarca LF, Bayona LM, Verpoorte R, et al. Broad range chemical profiling of natural deep eutectic solvent extracts using a high-performance thin layer chromatography–based method. Journal of Chromatography A. 2018; **1532**:198-207

[54] Liu KH, Lin HY, Thomas JL, Shih YP, Chen JT, Lee MH. Magnetic analogue-imprinted polymers for the extraction of ginsenosides from the *Panax ginseng* callus. Industrial Crops and Products. 2021;**163**:113291

[55] Choi YE, Jeong JH, Shin CK. Hormone-independent embryogenic callus production from ginseng cotyledons using high concentrations of NH_4/NO_3 and progress towards bioreactor production. Plant Cell, Tissue and Organ Culture. 2003;**72**(3):229-235

[56] Yang DC, Yang KJ, Choi YE. Production of red ginseng specific ginsenosides (Rg2, Rg3, Rh1 and Rh2) from *Agrobacterium*—Transformed hairy roots of *Panax ginseng* by heat treatment. Journal of Photoscience. 2001;**8**:19-22

[57] Thanh NT, Murthy HN, Yu KW, Hahn EJ, Paek KY. Methyl jasmonate elicitation enhanced synthesis of ginsenoside by cell suspension cultures of *Panax ginseng* in 5-l balloon type bubble bioreactors. Applied Microbiology and Biotechnology. 2005; **67**(2):197-201

[58] Wang W, Zhao ZJ, Xu Y, Qian X, Zhong JJ. Efficient induction of ginsenoside biosynthesis and alteration of ginsenoside heterogeneity in cell cultures of *Panax notoginseng* by using chemically synthesized 2-hydroxyethyl jasmonate. Applied Microbiology and Biotechnology. 2006;**70**(3):298-307

[59] Han J, Zhong JJ. Effects of oxygen partial pressure on cell growth and ginsenoside and polysaccharide production in high density cell cultures of *Panax notoginseng*. Enzyme and Microbial Technology. 2003;**32**(3-4): 498-503

[60] Wang J, Gao WY, Zhang J, Zuo BM, Zhang LM, Huang LQ. Production of ginsenoside and polysaccharide by two-stage cultivation of *Panax quinquefolium* L. cells. In Vitro Cellular & Developmental Biology-Plant. 2012;**48**(1):107-112

[61] Kochan E, Chmiel A. Dynamics of ginsenoside biosynthesis in suspension culture of *Panax quinquefolium*. Acta physiologiae plantarum. 2011;**33**(3): 911-915

[62] Kochan EWA, Caban S, Szymańska G, Szymczyk PIOT, Lipert A, Kwiatkowski P, et al. Ginsenoside content in suspension cultures of *Panax quinquefolium* L. cultivated in shake flasksand stirred-tank bioreactor. In: Annales Universitatis Mariae Curie-Sklodowska, sectio C–Biologia. Wydawnictwo Uniwersytetu Marii Curie-Skłodowskiej. Poland: Medical University of Lodz; 2017

[63] Thanh NT, Anh HT, Yoeup PK. Effects of macro elements on biomass and ginsenoside production in cell suspension culture of Ngoc Linh ginseng *Panax vietnamensis* Ha et Grushv. VNU Journal of Science: Natural Sciences and Technology. 2008;**24**(3):248-252

[64] Yu KW, Gao WY, Hahn EJ, Paek KY. Effects of macro elements and nitrogen source on adventitious root growth and ginsenoside production in ginseng (*Panax ginseng* CA Meyer). Journal of Plant Biology. 2001;**44**(4): 179-184

[65] Kim YS, Yeung EC, Hahn EJ, Paek KY. Combined effects of phytohormone, indole-3-butyric acid, and methyl jasmonate on root growth and ginsenoside production in adventitious root cultures of *Panax ginseng* CA Meyer. Biotechnology Letters. 2007;**29**(11):1789-1792

[66] Kim YS, Hahn EJ, Murthy HN, Paek KY. Effect of polyploidy induction on biomass and ginsenoside accumulations

in adventitious roots of ginseng. Journal of Plant Biology. 2004;**47**(4):356-360

[67] Yu KW, Gao W, Hahn EJ, Paek KY. Jasmonic acid improves ginsenoside accumulation in adventitious root culture of *Panax ginseng* CA Meyer. Biochemical Engineering Journal. 2002; **11**(2-3):211-215

[68] Jeong CS, Murthy HN, Hahn EJ, Lee HL, Paek KY. Inoculum size and auxin concentration influence the growth of adventitious roots and accumulation of ginsenosides in suspension cultures of ginseng (*Panax ginseng* CA Meyer). Acta physiologiae plantarum. 2009;**31**(1): 219-222

[69] Sivakumar G, Yu KW, Paek KY. Production of biomass and ginsenosides from adventitious roots of *Panax ginseng* in bioreactor cultures. Engineering in Life Sciences. 2005;**5**(4):333-342

[70] Yu KW, Hahn EJ, Paek KY. Effects of NH_4^+: NO_3^- Ratio and Ionic Strength on Adventitious Root Growth and Ginsenoside Production in Bioreactor Culture of *Panax ginseng* CA Meyer. Acta Horticulturae. 2001;**560**(49):259-262

[71] Jeong CS, Chakrabarty D, Hahn EJ, Lee HL, Paek KY. Effects of oxygen, carbon dioxide and ethylene on growth and bioactive compound production in bioreactor culture of ginseng adventitious roots. Biochemical Engineering Journal. 2006;**27**(3):252-263

[72] Yu Y, Zhang WB, Li XY, Piao XC, Jiang J, Lian ML. Pathogenic fungal elicitors enhance ginsenoside biosynthesis of adventitious roots in *Panax quinquefolius* during bioreactor culture. Industrial Crops and Products. 2016;**94**:729-735

[73] Kim OT, Yoo NH, Kim GS, Kim YC, Bang KH, Hyun DY, et al. Stimulation of Rg3 ginsenoside biosynthesis in ginseng

hairy roots elicited by methyl jasmonate. Plant Cell, Tissue and Organ Culture (PCTOC). 2013;**112**(1):87-93

[74] Mallol A, Cusidó RM, Palazón J, Bonfill M, Morales C, Piñol MT. Ginsenoside production in different phenotypes of *Panax ginseng* transformed roots. Phytochemistry. 2001;**57**(3):365-371

[75] Woo SS, Song JS, Lee JY, In DS, Chung HJ, Liu JR, et al. Selection of high ginsenoside producing ginseng hairy root lines using targeted metabolic analysis. Phytochemistry. 2004;**65**(20): 2751-2761

[76] Yu KW, Gao WY, Son SH, Paek KY. Improvement of ginsenoside production by jasmonic acid and some other elicitors in hairy root culture of ginseng (*Panax ginseng* CA Meyer). In Vitro Cellular & Developmental Biology-Plant. 2000;**36**(5):424-428

[77] Kim OT, Bang KH, Kim YC, Hyun DY, Kim MY, Cha SW. Upregulation of ginsenoside and gene expression related to triterpene biosynthesis in ginseng hairy root cultures elicited by methyl jasmonate. Plant Cell, Tissue and Organ Culture (PCTOC). 2009;**98**(1):25-33

[78] Kochan E, Szymczyk P, Kuźma Ł, Lipert A, Szymańska G. Yeast extract stimulates ginsenoside production in hairy root cultures of American ginseng cultivated in shake flasks and nutrient sprinkle bioreactors. Molecules. 2017;**22**(6):880

[79] Kochan E, Szymczyk P, Kuźma Ł, Szymańska G. Nitrogen and phosphorus as the factors affecting ginsenoside production in hairy root cultures of *Panax quinquefolium* cultivated in shake flasks and nutrient sprinkle bioreactor. Acta Physiologiae Plantarum. 2016;**38**(6):1-13

[80] Kochan E, Balcerczak E, Lipert A, Szymańska G, Szymczyk P. Methyl jasmonate as a control factor of the synthase squalene gene promoter and ginsenoside production in American ginseng hairy root cultured in shake flasks and a nutrient sprinkle bioreactor. Industrial Crops and Products. 2018;**115**: 182-193

[81] Kochan E, Szymańska G, Szymczyk P. Effect of sugar concentration on ginsenoside biosynthesis in hairy root cultures of *Panax quinquefolium* cultivated in shake flasks and nutrient sprinkle bioreactor. Acta Physiologiae Plantarum. 2014;**36**(3):613-619

[82] Kochan E, Królicka A, Chmiel A. Growth and ginsenoside production in *Panax quinquefolium* hairy roots cultivated in flasks and nutrient sprinkle bioreactor. Acta Physiologiae Plantarum. 2012;**34**(4):1513-1518

[83] Ha LT, Pawlicki-Jullian N, Pillon-Lequart M, Boitel-Conti M, Duong HX, Gontier E. Hairy root cultures of *Panax vietnamensis*, a promising approach for the production of ocotillol-type ginsenosides. Plant Cell, Tissue and Organ Culture (PCTOC). 2016;**126**(1): 93-103

[84] Choi YH, Verpoorte R. Metabolomics: What you see is what you extract. Phytochemical Analysis. 2014; **25**(4):289-290

Chapter 3

Ginseng: Pharmacological Action and Phytochemistry Prospective

Shuchi Dave Mehta, Priyanka Rathore and Gopal Rai

Abstract

Ginseng, the root of Panax species is a well-known conventional and perennial herb belonging to Araliaceae of various countries China, Korea, and Japan that is also known as the king of all herbs and famous for many years worldwide. It is a short underground rhizome that is associated with the fleshy root. Pharmacognostic details of cultivation and collection with different morphological characters are discussed. Phytocontent present is saponins glycosides, carbohydrates, polyacetylenes, phytosterols, nitrogenous substances, amino acids, peptides, vitamins, volatile oil, minerals, and enzymes details are discussed. The main focusing of the bioactive constituent of ginseng is ginsenosides are triterpenoid saponin glycosides having multifunctional pharmacological activities including anticancer, anti-inflammatory, antimicrobial, antioxidant and many more will be discussed. Ginseng is helpful in the treatment of microbial infection, inflammation, oxidative stress, diabetes, and obesity. Nanoparticles and nanocomposite film technologies had developed in it as novel drug delivery for cancer, inflammation, and neurological disorder. Multifaceted ginseng will be crucial for future development. This chapter review pharmacological, phytochemical, and pharmacognostic studies of this plant.

Keywords: Ginseng, ginsenosides, pharmacological, phytochemistry

1. Introduction

About 3.3 billion people in communities of less developed and even developed countries employ medicinal plants for the treatment and prevention of various diseases in their daily routine. Medicinal plant can be defined as the plant which contains metabolites that can be utilized for therapeutic indications or can be utilized for the synthesis of synthetic drugs. These plants are used in the indigenous system of medicine having no sufficient scientific predictions to confirm their therapeutic efficacy. Every medicinal plant consists of a variety of constituents that are involved in the synthesis and development of new and different kinds of the drug in the medicinal field.

Over 2000 years, China, Korea, and Siberia are major countries where ginseng was used as traditional medicine and commercial cultivation on a minor scale was in Germany, France, Holland, and England. the word ginseng i.e. Jen Sheng is originated from a Chinese word meaning 'man-herb' whereas the word Panax means 'all heal' in Greek which is a powerful plant that can all and any type of disease. **Figure 1** showing Ginseng a man root. It is commonly named as 'man root' due to the likeness of a man showing pharmacological uses of the whole body. In 1596, the Compendium of Materia Medica founded by Li Shizen discussed Ginseng as a "superior tonic" as compared to other herbal remedies. The usage of ginseng

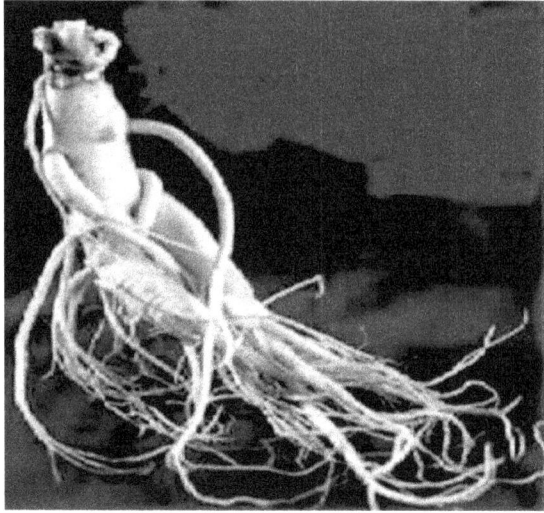

Figure 1.
Ginseng a man root.

is worldwide which is entitled as the most popular herbal remedy. It belongs to the genus Panax, the various species include *Panax quinquefolius*, *Panax ginseng*, and *Panax notoginseng* where their common names are American ginseng, Korean ginseng, and South China ginseng. The other species include *Panax japonicas*, *Panax vietnamensis*, *Panax pseudoginseng* All the species are regarded as wild where *Panax ginseng* is mostly cultivated.

2. Cultivation, collection, and preparation with morphological characters

These plants are cultivated in Northern Hemisphere countries mostly in China, Japan, Korea, United States, and Canada which requires a relatively cooler climate with temperatures between 0 and 25°C with loamy rich soil, well-drained land, and no direct sunlight, the shades are preferred. The height of the plant is 6 to 18 inches with greenish-yellow corollas with 15–30 flowers where light red, pear-shaped, globular fruits having 2 seeds.

Roots are thickened subcylindrical fleshy after drying the size is 25 cm long having 0.7–2.5 cm diameter, with 2–5 big branches where the outer surface is spirally wrinkled longitudinally with root scars.

The outer surface color differs in various varieties i.e., yellowish-white for Chinese and *Panax quinquefolius* and *Panax notoginseng* whereas yellowish-brown color for *Panax ginseng*. The taste is sweetish, mucilaginous and bitter sometimes where odor is slightly aromatic. The number of leaf scar in rhizome gives sign of age of plant. The yellowish-brown internal surface which is scattered with bark and wood containing brownish-red resin and oil [1, 2].

2.1 Plantation of ginseng seeds

After 3–6 years, either in autumn or summer season the roots are separated very carefully from plants due to presence of pest. For the purpose of avoidance of pest infection, the roots are sterilized and prepared. **Figure 2** showing plantation of ginseng.

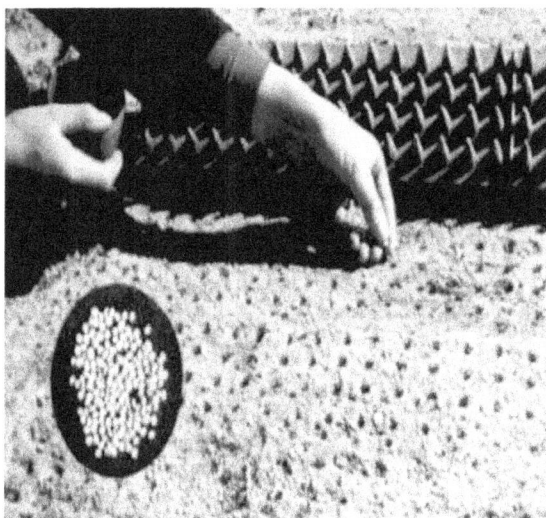

Figure 2.
Plantation of ginseng.

The method of preparation is different for white ginseng and red ginseng. In China, white ginseng' surface skin is removed by peeling and then dried and stored carefully for 12–15 months with less decrease of ginsenoside contents whereas in Korea, red ginseng is sterilized by steam sterilization method at a temperature of 120–130°C for about 3 hours which as a result saponin content is increased and can be stored for 2–3 years with no decrease of photo content.

2.2 Plants parts used

Root, Rhizomes, Leaves, Stem [3], flower bud [4].

2.3 Traditional uses

For more than a thousand years, ginseng was used as traditional herbal medicine as a healer of every type of disease. It was considered the best medicine for main fatigue and spiritlessness [5]. In traditional Chinese medicine, it was used for the treatment of heart and blood vessel disorder and also to make people feel calmer. In the ayurvedic system of medicine, traditionally ginseng was utilized as a cardioprotective, anticancer, and also as antioxidant.

3. Ginseng phytoconstituents

The classification of ginseng's phytochemistry consists of more than 200 chemical entities from ginseng species. The various groups of phytoconstituents include saponins glycosides, carbohydrates, polyacetylenes, phytosterols, nitrogenous substances, amino acids, peptides, vitamins, volatile oil, minerals, and enzymes.

3.1 Saponins

Saponins are the bioorganic glycoside having at least one glycosidic linkage at C3 between aglycone and sugar chain. On hydrolysis of saponin, molecule converts to glycone moiety i.e. glucose, pentose, galactose, maltose, fructose, or methyl pentose and aglycone moiety (sapogenin). The sapogenin can be classified as triterpenoid, steroid, alkaloid glycosides. Ginseng's saponins are usually known as ginsenosides which were named by Japanese workers whereas panxosides were named by Russian workers.

The ginsenosides are considered as the main constituents of ginseng having different pharmacological activities such as anti-fatigue, anti-cancer, anti-aging, anti-oxidant, anti-hyperglycemic, anti-obesity, and many more in ginseng root, berry, leaf, and stem. The basic structure of ginsenosides consists of a steroid nucleus with seventeen carbon atoms arranged in four rings. On the position of the hydroxyl group on carbon-20 shows are stereoisomers where every ginsenoside have at least 2 (carbon-3 and -20) or 3 (carbon-3, −6, and − 20) hydroxyl groups, which are free or bound to monomeric, dimeric, or trimeric sugars. Total gensenosides can be classified as oleanane, dammarane and ocotillol types. Ginsenoside Ro is an oleanane type whereas Gensenoside-Ral-3, G-Rbl-2, and G-Rh2 are dammarane type are subclassified into two types i.e., protopanaxadiols and protopanaxatriols. Pseudoginsenosides F11 and its derivatives such as makonoside-Rs are representative of ocotillol type ginsenosides [6]. Ginsenosides Rb2, Rb3, and Rg1 are showed on root hair, root and leaf whereas ginsenosides Rb3 and Rh1 were present in large amounts, and ginsenosides Rb1 and Rc were found in large amount main roots [4]. **Figure 3** showing various examples of ginsenosides. The pharmacological response of each ginsenoside is dependent on the type, position, and glycone moieties attached by the glycosidic bond at C-3, C-6, and C-20 positions. Among Panax species, more than 100 ginsenosides are isolated. More than 200 ginsenosides have been isolated and identified. The pharmacological effects include anti-electroconvulsive, memory enhancer, cardiac cell protector, coronary vascular dysfunction, antioxidant, antidiabetic, antiobesity, anti-foot and mouth disease, antiaging, antiulcer, antifatigue, and many more.

The bioavailability of ginsenosides is very poor. The absorption of ginsenosides in the intestinal mucosa is energy-dependent. The biliary excretion in active transport results in a shortage of its biological half-life and lower systemic exposure level [3, 7–9].

3.2 Carbohydrates

Among carbohydrates, the polysaccharides have considered highest content in the ginseng, which are classified into two parts according to their monosaccharide's structure i.e. ginseng starch like glucans and ginseng pectin. Neutral and acid polysaccharides are present in ginseng. These polysaccharides attribute pharmacological activity as immunomodulating, antioxidant, anti-depressant anticancer, anti-inflammatory, and antiproliferative activities by playing a vital role on nervous system disorders through regulation of signaling pathway, immune system and inflammatory response [10]. Two bioactive ginseng polysaccharides named GP50-dHR and GP50eHR showed antidiarrheal effects [11].

3.3 Amino acid

Organic compounds containing carboxyl and amine groups are known as amino acids. The concentration of amino acid in ginseng is large which is useful in human health that is applied in pharmaceutical and food applications. All the basic, acidic, and neutral amino acid including histidine, lysine, arginine, aspartic acid, glutamic acid, serine, alanine, glycine, proline, valine, tyrosine, leucine, and threonine plays as the major content of ginseng [12].

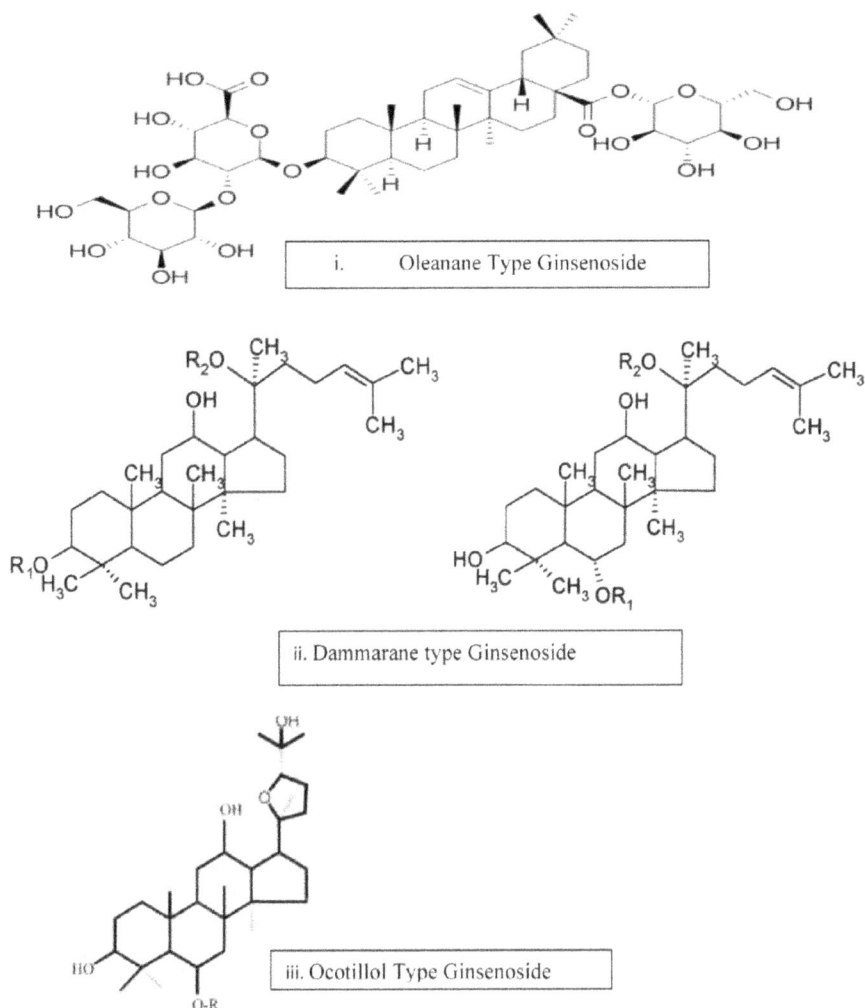

i.   Oleanane Type Ginsenoside

ii. Dammarane type Ginsenoside

iii. Ocotillol Type Ginsenoside

Figure 3.
Examples of Ginsenosides.

3.4 Polyacetylenes

The organic polymer with the repeating unit of polymerization of acetylene is known as polyacetylene. The total amount of polyacetylene in ginseng was reported as 0.020–0.073%. The anti-proliferative effect was reported in bioactive panaxynol and panaxydol, major polyacetylene in *Panax ginseng* Meyer roots using MTT assay viability method [13]. Ginsenoyne C is polyacetylene in *Panax Ginseng* showed anti-inflammatory through regulating phosphorylation of extracellular regulated kinases signaling [14].

3.5 Volatile oil

The pharmacological effects, qualities, and chemical content of volatile oil are varied to species to species of ginseng. More than 369 volatile oil compounds are identified in the ginseng species. Heterocycles, aldehydes, fatty acids, sesquiterpenoids, sesquiterpene hydrocarbon, alkane hydrocarbons, and fatty acid ester. Reported sesquiterpenoid includes bicyclogermacrene, calarene, (E)-β-farnesene, β-phellandrene, α-humulene where sesquiterpene hydrocarbon includes (E)-caryophyllene, aromadendrene, β-farnesene, α- neoclovene, β-neoclovene, bicyclogeracrene, α-panasinsene, β- panasinsene, ginsenol, panasinsenol A, panasinsenol B [15–17].

4. Pharmacological potential

Ginseng is considered a miracle source of multifaceted pharmacological activities such as anti-inflammatory, anticancer, antifungal, antibacterial, antiviral, immune-booster, antidiabetic, and antioxidant activities. **Figure 2** is showing various pharmacological uses of ginseng. The bioactive of ginseng has the power of interaction with membrane-bound ion channels, cell membranes, and extracellular and intracellular receptors which as consequences causes alteration at the transcriptional level. The extracts of Ginseng had shown protective effects on hepatocytes and liver injury. **Figure 4** showing Ginseng Pharmacological Potential. Previously demonstrated that both neurotrophic effects in learning and memory enhancement and also cause neuroprotective action for prevention of neuron degeneration [18–20].

4.1 Anti-inflammatory activity

Inflammation is an uncontrolled response that is the result of disorders including metabolic disorder, autoimmune diseases, cardiovascular disorder, or allergies; on the other hand, it is a response of our body to hazardous stimuli such as injury to tissues. For the treatment of suppressing and controlling inflammatory crisis various steroids, nonsteroids anti-inflammatory, and immunosuppressant are utilized. The inflammatory responses are classified as acute inflammation and chronic inflammation. Acute inflammation is for 7 days or a week whereas chronic inflammation extends for the past four weeks. During inflammation, cytokines are produced by Th1 cells (IL-2, interferon [IFN]-γ, TNF-α, and so on) will be decreased by Th2 cells releasing IL-4, IL-6, IL-10 and transforming growth factor-β. The mutual balance between Th1 and Th2 responses in inflammation immediately attenuate acute inflammation conditions back to normal whereas various conditions with imbalanced Th1/Th2 responses result in chronic inflammation [21].

Ginseng has suggested anti-inflammatory activity which was proven by various in vivo, in vitro, and clinical studies. Gensenosides Rb1, Rg1, Rg3, Re, Rd., Rh1, Rc, Rf, Rg5, Rg6, Rh3, Rk1, Ro, and Rz1 have been reported as anti-inflammatory responses due to negative regulation of pro-inflammatory cytokine expressions (TNF-α, IL-1β, and IL-6) and enzyme expressions in M1-polarized macrophages and microglia [22]. Ginsenosides Re and Rp1 can suppress the NF-κB signaling pathway whereas ginsenosides Rc inhibits macrophage-derived cytokines. Clinical studies concluded a 38% higher more survival rate for patients who took ginseng as compared to patients who had not taken ginseng [21]. Extract of *P. ginseng* berry calyx (Pg-C-EE) reported an anti-inflammatory mechanism through the expression of TNF-α, iNOS, COX-2 in lipopolysaccharide-activated macrophages and through NO production [23].

4.2 Anti-cancer activity

According to the world health organization, cancer is considered the second leading cause of death globally an estimated 9.6 million deaths or one in six deaths, in 2018. Cervical, thyroid, lung, colorectal, and breast cancer are common cancer

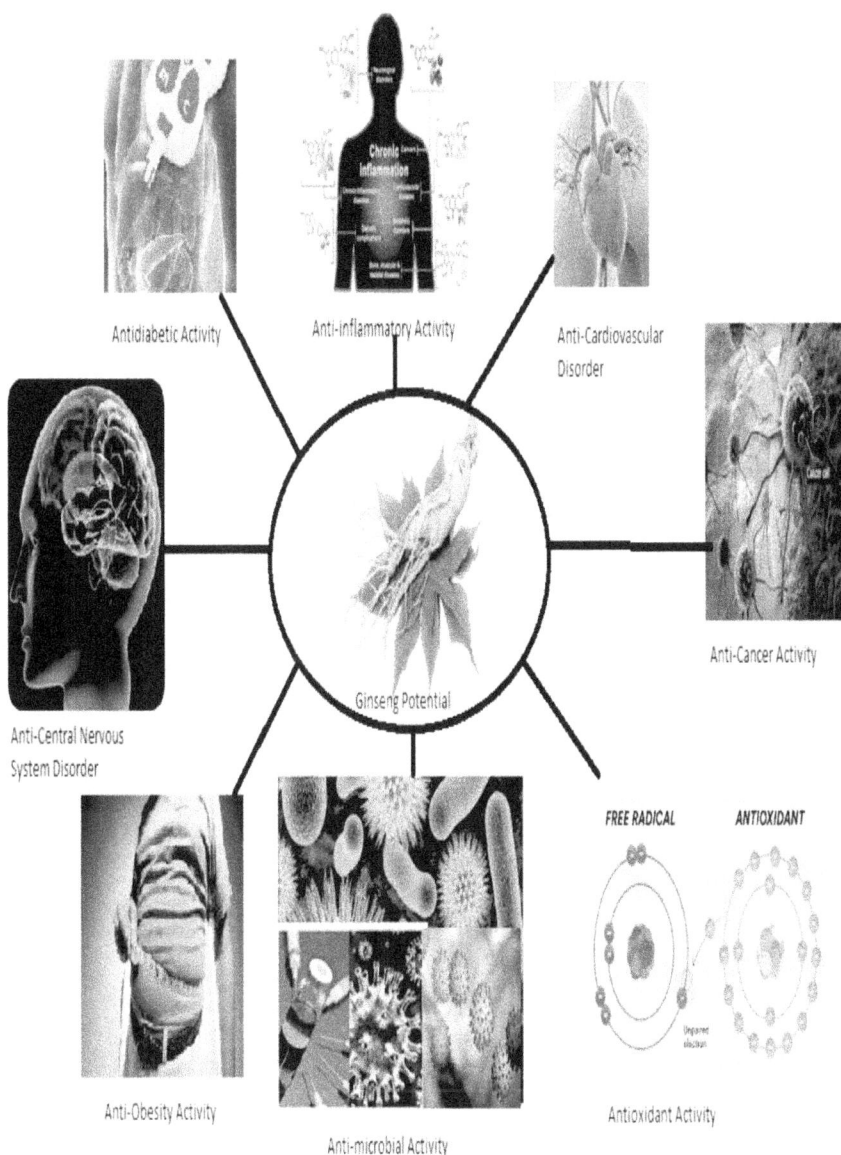

Figure 4.
Ginseng pharmacological potential.

diseases in women whereas stomach, liver, prostate, lung, and liver cancer are common cancer in men. Cancer can be defined as the growth of abnormal cells in uncontrolled conditions in almost any organ or tissue of the body, if beyond their usual boundaries then goes inside adjoining parts of the body and spread to other organs. At metastasizing process, results in cancer death. Cancer can be prevented by implementing evidence-based strategies by avoiding the risk factors use of tobacco, use of alcohol, less consumption of fruits and vegetables. For the treatment of cancer, chemotherapy is the most common therapy for treatment. Administration of chemotherapeutic agents as result gives a reduction in bone density and immunosuppression.

For many years, natural products have been a good source of agents for treating cancer and plants played a huge role in anti-cancer product development. Ginseng is a universal herb that is utilized for the prevention and treatment of cancer. It has been acting as a chemopreventive and also used to improve the quality of life among patients with cancer [24, 25]. Ginseng as an herbal drug is consumed and mentioned in the Pharmacopieas formulation in various countries like United Kingdom, China, Japan, France, Austria, and Germany. In Western Europe and Asian countries, it is commonly utilized as a combinational drug to improve cancer chemotherapy. Ginseng is responsible for the inhibition of the growth of human cancer cells of prostate cancer, lung cancer, and colon cancer. **Figure 5** is showing Ginsenoside anticancer activity.

4.3 Anti-cancer activity

According to the world health organization, cancer is considered the second leading cause of death globally an estimated 9.6 million deaths or one in six deaths, in 2018. Cervical, thyroid, lung, colorectal, and breast cancer are common cancer diseases in women whereas stomach, liver, prostate, lung, and liver cancer are common cancer in men. Cancer can be defined as the growth of abnormal cells in uncontrolled conditions in almost any organ or tissue of the body, if beyond

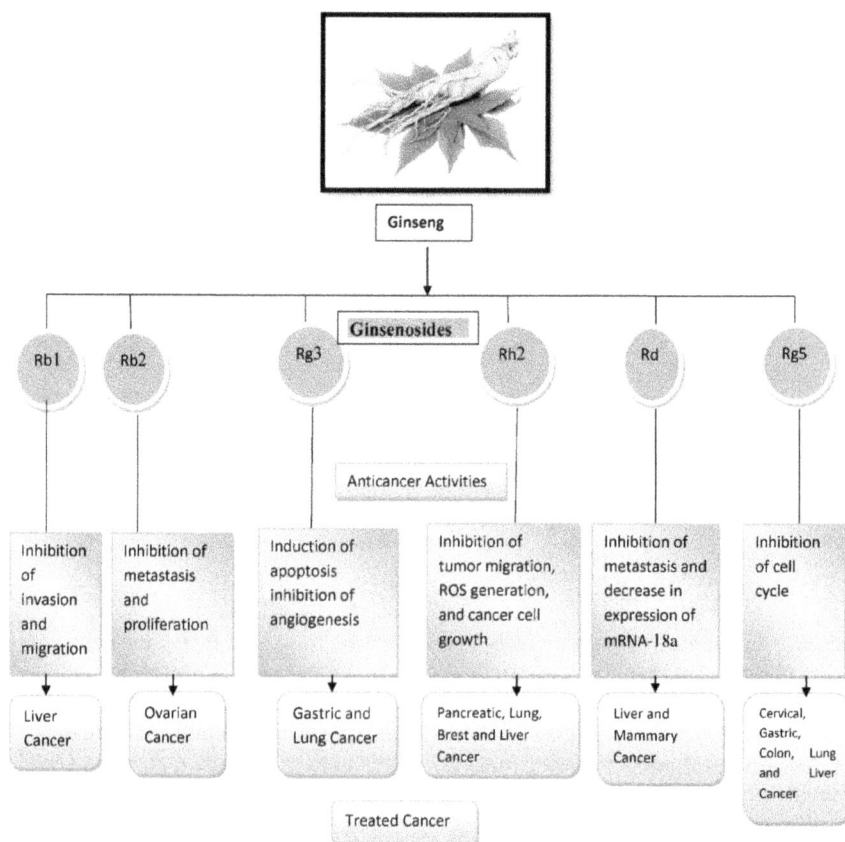

Figure 5.
Ginsenoside anticancer activity.

their usual boundaries then goes inside adjoining parts of the body and spread to other organs. At metastasizing process, results in cancer death. Cancer can be prevented by implementing evidence-based strategies by avoiding the risk factors use of tobacco, use of alcohol, less consumption of fruits and vegetables. For the treatment of cancer, chemotherapy is the most common therapy for treatment. Administration of chemotherapeutic agents as result gives a reduction in bone density and immunosuppression.

For many years, natural products have been a good source of agents for treating cancer and plants played a huge role in anti-cancer product development. Ginseng is a universal herb that is utilized for the prevention and treatment of cancer. It has been acting as a chemopreventive and also used to improve the quality of life among patients with cancer [24, 25]. Ginseng as an herbal drug is consumed and mentioned in the Pharmacopieas formulation in various countries like United Kingdom, China, Japan, France, Austria, and Germany. In Western Europe and Asian countries, it is commonly utilized as a combinational drug to improve cancer chemotherapy. Ginseng is responsible for the inhibition of the growth of human cancer cells of prostate cancer, lung cancer, and colon cancer. **Figure 5** is showing Ginsenoside anticancer activity.

The anticancer action is by modulation of diverse signaling pathways, including regulation of cell proliferation mediators (cyclins and CDKs), growth factors (c-myc, vascular endothelial growth factor, and EGFR), tumor suppressor (p53 and p21), cell mediators (Bcl-2, caspases, Bcl-xl, death receptors), inflammatory response molecules (COX-2 and NFκB), protein kinase (JNK, Akt, and AMP-activated protein kinase) It acts on its cellular and molecular targets through various pathways by inhibiting the tumor by regulation of the cell cycle and inhibition of angiogenesis and invasion [26].

Ginseng extract can induce chemosensitization of the conventional anticancer agent through multidrug resistance (MDR-1) associated protein. Ginseng had also shown a reduction of drug-induced toxicity when used in combination with anticancer drug for example ginsenosides Rh4 and Rk3 reduces the cisplatin-induced nephrotoxicity in dose dependant level where the reason and structure–activity relationship with other ginsenosides are remained to be studied by Baek *et al.* [27, 28].

In clinical studies, Ginseng is acting as a tonic in combination with chemotherapy which concluded that ginseng with the other anticancer drug, for example navebine, Vinorelbine, enhances the short term therapeutic efficiency of lung cancer where the study was conducted by 63 patients. The result showed an improvement in the patient's quality of life. Researchers are focusing on purified ginsenosides which gives the result to a rapid specific mechanism of action rather than using ginseng extract.

Ginseng polysaccharides are also reported as an anticancer agent which includes fractions such as WGPA-1-RG, WGPA-2-RG, WGPA-1-HG, WGPA-2-HG, WGPA-3-HG, and WGPA-4-HG that acts by regulating the immune response of host organisms whereas Ginseng pectin reported inhibiting the action of proteins linked with cancer progression [24].

4.4 Antimicrobial activity

Antimicrobial activity was derived from the Greek words anti-meaning against, mikros meaning little, and bios meaning life which can be defined as the activity against the growth of microorganisms or by their killing. The microorganisms include bacterial, fungi, parasites or viruses. Antiviral activity is defined as the action of killing a virus or suppression of its ability to replicate and inhibition of the virus for multiplication and reproduction. It is used in the treatment of infectious disease caused by a virus where the virus responsible for the disease include influenza, herpes simplex type 1 and type 2, herpes zoster, viral hepatitis, encephalitis, infectious mononucleosis, HIV/AIDS, and many more. Viruses are nucleic acid i.e. DNA or RNA and a protein coat.

Novel antiviral formulation therapies and vaccines are in recent progress of research scientists which supported to prevent and shorten the duration of the extremity of viral infection. Due to the continuous growth of new infection of the Ebola virus and respiratory syndrome coronavirus, it is compulsory to develop advanced novel therapeutic approaches. The main problem in the development of novel antiviral agent is mutation process in the viral mutation that as result in drug resistance and immune evasion. Recently the development of novel antiviral formulation has the target to develop broad-spectrum antiviral and immunomodulators which improve and inhibit the host resistance to the viral infection In large population infection, vaccination is the main measure of treatment of disease [29, 30].

In vitro and in vivo antiviral activity of Panax Korean red ginseng extract was determined on respiratory syncytial virus infection (RSV) which as a result showed improved the survival of human lung epithelial cells against RSV infection and also inhibited RSV replication by suppressing the expression of RSV-induced inflammatory cytokine genes and also enhanced level of interferon-γ producing dendritic cells which are subsequent to RSV infection [30].

Antiviral activity of fermented *Panax ginseng* extracts against a broad spectrum of Influenza viruses (H1N1, H3N2, H5N1, and H7N9) in genetically diverse mouse models was investigated. Antiviral protection was observed due to more components of saponins of fermented ginseng extracts against influenza viruses than nonfermented ginseng extract. For the development of a new vaccine and new antiviral drug against influenza viruses, the Panax notoginseng root was studied where both in vitro and in vivo analysis was investigated. The Panax notoginseng root decreased influenza A virus-induced mortality by 90% and also increased the NK cell activity of mouse splenocytes [31].

Antifungal is an agent for the treatment and prevention of fungal infections which selectively eliminates fungal pathogen from a host with minimal toxicity to the host. Fungi examples are yeast, *Candida albicans, molds, Xanthoriaparietina, Amanita phalloides, Polyphagus euglena, Gigaspora gigantean* and many more. Korean red ginseng containing saponin as ginsenosides were reported as having antifungal effects against *Candida albicans*. The result was concluded that ginsenosides antifungal activity by disrupting the structure of cell membrane were awaited for further clinical investigation [32].

The root of ginseng, Notoginseng was investigated antifungal activities against *Epidermophyton floccosum, Trichophyton rubrum*, and *Trichophyton mentagrophytes*. The mechanism of antifungal activity was to find out which was due to interaction with the fungal cell membrane and damages the integrity of the membrane. The result concluded that notoginseng saponin can used for the treatment of ringworm [33].

Antibacterial and antifungal effect of ginseng powder on gram-positive, gram-negative, and *Staphylococcus aureus, Pseudomonas aeruginosa, Escherichia coli, Enterococcus faecalis* and *Candida albicans* as fungus was investigated by disc diffusion method showed significant zone inhibition [34].

4.5 Antioxidant activity

Antioxidant activity is the limitation and inhibition of nutrient oxidation by restraining oxidative chain reactions. Herbal antioxidants prevent destructive processes caused by oxidative stress by stabilizing or deactivate free radicals before they attack targets in a biological cell. Cancer, diabetes, inflammation, senile dementia, asthma, liver damage, and many other diseases are closely related to free radicals. Free radicals are originated from various sources such as pollution, alcohol, tobacco, smoking, pesticides, phagocytic cells etc. In vitro and in vivo antioxidant effect of *Panax ginseng* showed higher free radical scavenging activity power than white and red ginseng which was due to the presence of higher content of total saponin, phenolic, and flavonoids. The antioxidant activity analyzes by free radical scavenging activity assay and reducing power assay method, lipid peroxidation, antioxidant enzyme activity models [35].

The antioxidant effect of *Panax Ginseng* was studied on healthy volunteers of 82 participants of which 21 men and 61 women were investigated where Serum level of reactive oxygen species (ROS), malondialdehyde (MDA), total antioxidant capacity (TAC), the activities of catalase, superoxide dismutase (SOD), glutathione reductase (GSH-Rd), and peroxidase (GSH-Px), and total glutathione content were determined. The healthy volunteers confirmed the antioxidant potential of *P. ginseng*. *P. quinquefolius* containing ginsenosides analyzed affinity DPPH-stable free radical, metal chelation, and hydroxyl free radicals for characterization of antioxidant effect [36].

5. Novel formulation development

Ginseng as a supertonic herbal drug should be in novel approaches that get rid of the limitation of the conventional drug. Novel approaches will help in increase of bioavailability, minimize drug physical and chemical degradation and loss, prevention of harmful side-effects, protecting toxicity and enhancement stability. This will help to overcome problems associated with herbal medicine. Herbal Novel drug delivery includes nanoparticles, liposomes, phytosomes, nanoemulsion, microsphere, transferosomes, nanocapsules and ethosomes are reported using extract and marker Nanoparticles and nanocomposite technology of ginseng had reported previously [37, 38].

A novel multifunctional liposome system was developed in a combination of three ginsenosides with paclitaxel using the thin-film hydration method. Antitumor activity was analyzed by GC, MTT, cell cycle, and apoptosis assays method. The result concluded that ginseng liposome was acting as tumor-targeting therapy with dual effect as chemotherapy adjuvant and functional membrane material [39]. Nanoginseng showed better antitumor activity and high drug load efficiency and capacity, excellent biocompatibility with reduced damage to normal tissues [40]. Nanocapsulated red ginseng extract using bioactive coating materials chitosan enhanced antithrombotic activities by both in-vitro and ex vivo platelet aggregation assay method [41]. Phytosome *Panax ginseng* containing ginsenosides acting as nutraceutical and immunomodulator elevated superoxide dismutase, glutathione peroxidase, and glutathione reductase activities. Commercial product of phytosome as Ginseng PhytosomeTM is in market.

6. Conclusion

The traditional system of medicine including the Chinese system of medicine and Ayurvedic system of medicine already mentioned ginseng as man herb acting as a supertonic which is used for the treatment of all type of disease cancer, cardiovascular disorder, impotence, diabetes, palpitation, insomnia, hyperdynamic, anorexia, and many more. Unique cultivation and collection techniques are discussed. More than 200 phytochemical are reported where main classes include saponins glycosides, carbohydrates, polyacetylenes, phytosterols, nitrogenous substances, amino acids, peptides, vitamins, volatile oil, minerals, and enzymes. The miracle ginseng consist of anti-inflammatory, anticancer, antifungal, antibacterial, antiviral, immune- booster, antidiabetic, and antioxidant activities pharmacological actions of which latest anticancer, anti-inflammatory, antimicrobial, and antioxidant pharmacological activities is discussed where not only in vivo and in vitro studies is discussed but also clinical trial is highlighted. Novel formulation phytosome, nanocapsulated, nanoparticles for cancer, inflammation, and neurological disorder developed to enhance bioavailability and target delivery of drug. It can be concluded that focusing the herb in research and development of the pharmaceutical industry in private and government agencies in future development would be beneficial and helpful to eliminate the toxic effect of supertonic ginseng.

Author details

Shuchi Dave Mehta[1*], Priyanka Rathore[2] and Gopal Rai[1]

1 Guru Ramdas Khalsa Institute of Science and Technology (Pharmacy), Jabalpur, MP, India

2 Sagar Institute of Research and Technology Pharmacy, Bhopal, MP, India

*Address all correspondence to: shuchi1801@gmail.com

IntechOpen

References

[1] Natasya Trivena Rokot, Timothy Sean Kairupan, Kai-Chun Cheng, Joshua Runtuwene, Nova Hellen Kapantow, Marie Amitani, Akinori Morinaga, Haruka Amitani, Akihiro Asakawa, and Akio Inui; 'A Role of Ginseng and Its Constituents in the Treatment of Central Nervous System Disorders'; Evidence-Based Complementary and Alternative Medicine 2016; 2614742; 2016.

[2] Evans, W. C., Evans, D., and Trease, G. E.; Trease and Evans pharmacognosy; 2009; 16th edition; Edinburgh; New York: Saunders/Elsevier, PP-311-312

[3] Wang, H., Peng, D. & Xie, J. Ginseng leaf-stem: bioactive constituents and pharmacological functions; Chinese Medicine; 2009; 4, 20;https://doi.org/10.1186/1749-8546-4-20.

[4] Kang OJ, Kim JS. Comparison of Ginsenoside Contents in Different Parts of Korean Ginseng (Panax ginseng C.A. Meyer). PrevNutr Food Sci. 2016; 21 (4):389-392. doi:10.3746/pnf.2016. 21.4.389

[5] Kim JH. Pharmacological and medical applications of Panax ginseng and ginsenosides: a review for use in cardiovascular diseases. J Ginseng Res. 2018; 42(3) : 264-269. doi:10.1016/j.jgr.2017.10.004

[6] Kim JH, Yi YS, Kim MY, Cho JY. Role of ginsenosides, the main active components of Panax ginseng, in inflammatory responses and diseases; Journal of Ginseng Research; J Ginseng Res. 2017; 41(4):435-443.

[7] Jia L, Zhao Y. Current evaluation of the millennium phytomedicine--ginseng (I): etymology, pharmacognosy, phytochemistry, market and regulations. Curr Med Chem. 2009; 16(19); PP-2475-2484.

[8] Liu a Hanbing , Lu b Xiaoyan, Hu b Yang, Fan a Xiaohui,; Chemical constituents of *Panax ginseng* and Panax notoginseng explain why they differ in therapeutic efficacy; Pharmacological research;2020; 161; 105263.

[9] Lü JM, Yao Q, Chen C. Ginseng compounds: an update on their molecular mechanisms and medical applications. CurrVascPharmacol. 2009;7(3):293-302. doi:10.2174/157016109788340767

[10] Na Wang, Xianlei Wang, Mengjiao He, Wenxiu Zheng, Dongmei Qi, Yongqing Zhang, Chun-chao Han; Ginseng polysaccharides: A potential neuroprotective agent; Journal of Ginseng Research; Volume 45, Issue 2; 2021; P-211-217.

[11] Seung-HoonBaek, JinGyun Lee, Seo Young Park, Ok Nam Bae, Dong-Hyun Kim, and Jeong Hill Park; Pectic Polysaccharides from Panax ginseng as the Antirotavirus Principals in Ginseng; Biomacromolecules; 2010; 11 (8); 2044-2052

[12] Zhi Liu, Xin Wen, Chong-Zhi Wang, Wei Li, Wei-Hua Huang, Juan Xia, Chang-Chun Ruan, Chun-Su Yuan; Remarkable impact of amino acids on ginsenoside transformation from fresh ginseng to red ginseng; Journal of Ginseng Research; Volume 44, Issue 3; 2020; PP 424-434.

[13] Yeo CR, Yong JJ, Popovich DG. Isolation and characterization of bioactive polyacetylenes *Panax ginseng* Meyer roots; Journal Pharm Biomed Anal. 2017 May 30;139:148-155. doi: ayush10.1016/j.jpba.2017.02.054. Epub 2017 Mar 1. PMID: 28282601.

[14] Yup SS, Hyun SS, Mina L; Ginsenoyne C, a polyacetylene isolated from *Panax Ginseng* inhibit inflammatory mediators via regulating extracellular regulated kinases

signaling; Pharmacognosy Magazine;2018;14; 57; 358-362.

[15] In Hee Cho, Hyun Jeong Lee, and Young-Suk Kim; Journal of Agricultural and Food Chemistry; 2012; 60; (31), 7616-7622.

[16] Cho, I.H. Volatile compounds of ginseng (Panax sp.): a review.; J Korean Soc Appl Biol Chem; 2015;58, 67-75.

[17] Kim JS. Investigation of Phenolic, Flavonoid, and Vitamin Contents in Different Parts of Korean Ginseng (Panax ginseng C.A. Meyer). PrevNutr Food Sci. 2016; 21(3):263-270. doi:10.3746/pnf.2016.21.3.263

[18] Wee JJ, Mee Park K, Chung AS; Biological Activities of Ginseng and Its Application to Human Health; Herbal Medicine: Biomolecular and Clinical Aspects; 2011; 2nd edition; Chapter 8. Boca Raton (FL): CRC Press/Taylor & Francis; Available from: https://www. ncbi.nlm.nih.gov/books/NBK92776

[19] Yuan, Chun-Su, Huu Tung, Nguyen, Uto, Takuhiro, Morinaga, Osamu, Kim, Young Ho, Shoyama, Yukihiro; Pharmacological Effects of Ginseng on Liver Functions and Diseases: A Minireview; Evidence-Based Complementary and Alternative Medicine;2012; 2012/09/11; 173297; Hindawi Publishing Corporation.

[20] Zubair Ahmed Ratan, Mohammad Faisal Haidere, Yo Han Hong, Sang Hee Park, Jeong-Oog Lee, Jongsung Lee, Jae Youl Cho; Pharmacological potential of ginseng and its major component ginsenosides; Journal of Ginseng Research; 2021; 45;2; P-199-210.

[21] Park J and Cho JY; Anti-inflammatory effects of ginsenosides from *Panax ginseng* and their structural analogs; African Journal of Biotechnology; 2009; Vol. 8 (16); P 3682-3690.

[22] Im D-S. Pro-Resolving Effect of Ginsenosides as an Anti-Inflammatory Mechanism of Panax ginseng. Biomolecules. 2020; 10(3):444.

[23] Han S Y, Kim J, Kim E, Kim S H, Seo D, Kim J H, Shin S S, Cho J Y; AKT-targeted anti-inflammatory activity of *Panax ginseng* calyx ethanolic extract; Journal of Ginseng Research; 2018; 42(4); P-496-503.

[24] Chen S, Wang Z, Huang Y, O'Barr SA, Wong RA, Yeung S, Chow MS. Ginseng and anticancer drug combination to improve cancer chemotherapy: a critical review. Evidence Based Complement Alternative Med. 2014; 168940. doi: 10.1155/2014/168940. Epub 2014 Apr 30. PMID: 24876866; PMCID: PMC4021740.

[25] Sun, M., Ye, Y., Xiao, L., Duan, X., Zhang, Y., & Zhang, H.; Anticancer effects of ginsenoside Rg3 (Review). International Journal of Molecular Medicine; 2017; 39; 507-518.

[26] Zuo, Zhong, Chen, Shihong, AU - Wang, Zhijun, Huang, Ying, O'Barr, Stephen A, Wong, Rebecca A, Yeung, Steven, Chow, Moses Sing Sum; Ginseng and Anticancer Drug Combination to Improve Cancer Chemotherapy: A Critical Review; Evidence-Based Complementary and Alternative Medicine; 2014; 2014/04/30; Hindawi Publishing Corporation; https://doi. org/10.1155/2014/168940.

[27] C. Choi, G. Kang, and Y. Min; Reversal of P-glycoprotein-mediated multidrug resistance by protopanaxatriol ginsenosides from Korean red ginseng; Planta Medica; 2003; 69; 3, PP-235-240,.

[28] S. H. Baek, X. L. Piao, U. J. Lee, H. Y. Kim, and J. H. Park, "Reduction of cisplatin-induced nephrotoxicity by ginsenosides isolated from processed ginseng in cultured renal tubular cells; Biological and Pharmaceutical Bulletin; 2006; 29;10; PP. 2051-2055,

[29] Im, Kyungtaek& Kim, Jisu& Min, Hyeyoung; Ginseng, the natural effectual antiviral: Protective effects of Korean Red Ginseng against viral infection; Journal of Ginseng Research; 2016; 40; PP 309-314.

[30] Lee JS, Ko EJ, Hwang HS, et al. Antiviral activity of ginseng extract against respiratory syncytial virus infection; International Journal of Molecular Medicine; 2014; 34(1):183-190.

[31] Choi, Jang-Gi and Jin, Young-Hee and Lee, Heeeun and Oh, Tae Woo and Yim, Nam-Hui and Cho, Won-Kyung and Ma, JinYeul; Protective Effect of Panax notoginseng Root Water Extract against Influenza A Virus Infection by Enhancing Antiviral Interferon-Mediated Immune Responses and Natural Killer Cell Activity; Frontiers in Immunology;2017;8;PP-1542.

[32] Sung WS, Lee DG. In vitro candidacidal action of Korean red ginseng saponins against *Candida albicans*. Biological Pharmaceutical Bulletin; 2008; 31(1); PP-139-142.

[33] Peng Xue, Xiushi Yang, XiaoyanSunab and Guixing Ren; Antifungal activity and mechanism of heattransformed ginsenosides from notoginseng against Epidermophyton floccosum, Trichophyton rubrum, and Trichophyton mentagrophytes; Royal Society of Chemistry Advances; 2017; 7; P-10939.a

[34] Meskini, Maryam & Mohammadbeigi, Maryam & Solati, Jalal & Alimoradi, Samira; Antibacterial and Antifungal Effect of Ginseng Powder; 2019; 11th International congress of Laboratory and clinic.

[35] Chung SI, Kang MY, Lee SC. In Vitro and In Vivo Antioxidant Activity of Aged Ginseng (*Panax ginseng*); Preventive Nutritive Food Science; 2016;21(1):PP-24-30.

[36] Kim HG, Yoo SR, Park HJ, et al. Antioxidant effects of *Panax ginseng* C.A. Meyer in healthy subjects: a randomized, placebo-controlled clinical trial.; Food Chemistry Toxicology; 2011;49(9); PP-2229-2235.

[37] Devi VK, Jain N, Valli KS. Importance of novel drug delivery systems in herbal medicines. Pharmacognosy Review; 2010;4(7): 27-31. doi:10.4103/0973-7847.65322

[38] Ajazuddin, S. Saraf; Applications of novel drug delivery system for herbal formulations; Fitoterapia; 2010; 81(7); PP 680-689.

[39] Hong C, Wang D, Liang J, Guo Y, Zhu Y, Xia J, Qin J, Zhan H, Wang J. Novel ginsenoside-based multifunctional liposomal delivery system for combination therapy of gastric cancer; Theranostics;2019; 9(15):4437-4449

[40] Dai, Lin & Zhu, Weiyan& Chuanling, Si & Lei, Jiandu; Nano-Ginseng" for enhanced cytotoxicity AGAINST cancer cells; International Journal of Molecular Sciences.; 2018; 19; PP 627.

[41] Eun Suh Kim, Ji-Soo Lee, and Hyeon Gyu Lee; Nanoencapsulation of Red Ginseng Extracts Using Chitosan with Polyglutamic Acid or Fucoidan for Improving Antithrombotic Activities; Journal of Agricultural and Food Chemistry; 2016; 64 (23), 4765-4771.

.

Chapter 4

Anti-Inflammatory Potential of Ginseng for Wound Healing

Dimple Sethi Chopra, Abhishek Gupta, Dhandeep Singh and Nirmal Singh

Abstract

The recovery of skin wounds is a complex biological process involving three basic mechanisms: inflammatory phase, re-epithelialization followed by granulation and tissue remodeling. The interactions between inflammatory cells, fibroblasts, and keratinocytes induce microenvironmental changes at the wound site. Tissue remodeling is initiated by matrix-producing proteins and protease enzymes and collagen fibers in the dermis. A saponin extracted from ginseng, known as ginsenoside, has been shown to accelerate neovascularization in burn wounds in mice. It also increases levels of vascular endothelial growth factor and interleukin (IL-β). IL-β accelerate wound healing by promoting accumulation of macrophages at skin wound sites. Saponins are major active constituents of ginseng. They contain many ginsenosides. The purified ginsenosides or the extracts of ginseng root have been reported to have beneficial effects on damaged skin. For instance, red ginseng root extract protected skin from acute UVB-irradiation. Ginsenoside F_1, an enzymatically modified derivative of the ginsenoside Rg_1, protected HaCaT against UVB-induced apoptosis. *Panax ginseng* root extract promotes type I collagen synthesis in human dermal fibroblasts (HDF) via the Smad activation pathway and exhibits antioxidant activity against free radicles including diphenyl-p-picrylhydrazyl treatment. In addition, ginsenoside Rb_1 promotes healing process of burn wound by enhancing angiogenesis. Among the various ginsenosides, ginsenoside Rb_1 has been found to most potent agent for wound healing.

Keywords: *Panax ginseng*, skin wound healing, total ginseng saponin, mice, ginsenoside Rd., wound-healing, cyclic AMP-dependent protein kinase, keratinocyte progenitor cells, human dermal fibroblasts

1. Introduction

A wound is disruption of barrier function of the skin which may result from a physical or chemical injury. Depending on time taken for healing process, it can be categorized as simple, acute wound and chronic wound. The human body has the potential to initiate wound healing process in order to replace the damaged cellular structures and tissue layers. This complex process is comprises of sequence of events starting from homeostasis, inflammation, proliferation/granulation leading to remodeling/maturation [1].

Acute wounds are characterized by minimal localized microbial infection and scab formation. Infiltration of immune cells leads to re-epithelialization, angiogenesis and fibroblast migration. If the immune system is unable to control the infection, microbial biofilm is formed leading to impaired wound healing. Chronic wounds are characterized by increased inflammatory process, lower oxygenation of the deep tissues due to fibrin cuffs formation, fibroblast senescence, impaired angiogenesis and re-epithelialization. Most chronic wounds are ulcers that are associated with ischemia, diabetes mellitus, venous stasis disease, or pressure [2, 3].

Wound care is a million-dollar global industry which determines the appropriate treatment to promote wound healing with minimal infections [4]. Several aspects of wound healing are encompassed in the management including, but not limiting to maintaining optimum moist environment at the wound site, infection control, treatments for deep seated tissue regeneration using stem cell therapy [4, 5]. Despite medical advancements in wound care, there is a mounting demand for alternative treatments from the clinical and economic perspective. It has been reported that chronic wounds affect 6.5 million people in the USA, and costs over US $25 billion each year. Alarmingly, the burden of chronic wounds is expected to rise due to global increases in vascular diseases, diabetes, obesity, metabolic syndrome, and the general aging of the population [6]. In ancient times, tribal people used plants to cure wounds. Even now, plants are considered as huge source of novel bioactive agents. It has been found that at present there are more than 450 plant species being extensively used for their wound healing ability, yet the search for novel wound healing agents from natural resources with minimal scaring is never ending [7].

There are numerous medicaments available to augment skin wound healing, disinfectants like ethyl alcohol, iodine, ether, ointments containing antibiotics and steroid hormones. Iodine based preparations and silver releasing agents have been used as antimicrobial agents to treat infected wounds. They target bacteria at cell membrane, cytoplasmic organelle, and nucleic acid level, thus minimizing bacterial resistance [8]. They can be used either alone or in conjunction with systemic antibiotics. Advanced silver dressings, aim to deliver sustained doses of silver to the wound [9, 10]. In addition to the microbicidal effect of silver on common wound contaminants, silver may also be effective against resistant strains like methicillin resistant *Staphylococcus aureus* (MRSA). Zinc, an antioxidant, used in a paste bandage is useful in treating infected leg ulcers. Phenytoin, applied topically, promotes wound healing by inhibiting the enzyme collagenase. It is effective in some low grade pressure ulcers and trophic ulcers due to leprosy. The possibility of systemic absorption and toxicity has limited its use. Analgesics are in great demand for treatment of ulcers. They may comprise of simple analgesics like NSAIDs or strong analgesics like opiates in case of severe pain. Tricyclic antidepressants (such as amitriptyline) or antiepileptic drugs (such as gabapentin) are drugs of choice for ulcers associated with neuropathic pain [11]. These agents provide preliminary relief but interfere with the normal healing process. They injure not only invading foreign organisms but also normal body cells. They can lead to emergence of resistant bacterial infection and hypersensitivity reactions. From ancient times, various natural substances have been widely used for wound healing [12].

The polyphenols in plant extracts are capable of neutralizing free radicals by combining with active oxygen [13]. A stable phenoxyl radical is formed when a polyphenolic compound combines with free radicals formed during the metabolic process. Superoxide, hydroxyl, lipid peroxyl, nitric oxide radicals, and peroxynitrites are the most common free radicals with which polyphenolic compounds usually combine. In wounds there is a high oxidative stress due to the activation of platelets, neutrophils, macrophages, lymphocytes and fibroblasts. The concentration of reactive oxygen species varies at different time points of the healing process [3]. This is further enhanced by infection from microbes. In such conditions, plant based polyphenol may assist in the healing process by modulating the concentrations of reactive oxygen species [14].

In case of burn wounds, coagulative necrosis is quite predominant resulting in scar formation after repair. Macrophages migrate to the injured area to kill invading organisms and produce cytokines that recruit other inflammatory cells that are responsible for cascade of inflammatory reactions. Angiogenesis at the injured area is vital in wound healing process. Moreover, growth factors and cytokines play crucial role in wound-healing process [15, 16]. Hypoxia induces cytokine and growth factor production from macrophages, keratinocytes, and fibroblasts. These include platelet-derived growth factor (PDGF), transforming growth factor (TGF-β), vascular endothelial growth factor (VEGF), tumor necrosis factor-α (TNF-α), and endothelin-1. They in turn promote cell proliferation, migration, chemotaxis and angiogenesis in wound healing [17]. Although, hypoxia stimulates wound healing such as the release of growth factors and angiogenesis, still oxygen is needed to sustain the healing process [18].

Hence, burn wound healing is a multiple step process, involving inflammatory phases such as monocyte migration, cytokine production, growth factors and angiogenesis during re-epithelialization. Preliminary experiments, reveal that total ginseng saponins isolated from Red Ginseng roots accelerated burn wound healing in mice. There are significant number of indications on wound healing effects of ginsenosides with diverse associated mechanisms, one such report is on skin regeneration by the ginsenoside Rd (discussed later in the chapter) isolated from ginseng leaves. GinsenosideRb_1 promotes burn wound healing process by enhancing angiogenesis [19].

2. Anatomical and physiological changes in wound bed

In mammals, wound healing is a rapid process involving cessation of bleeding from the wound, restoration of damaged tissues, moisture deposition around the wound to develop functional defense membrane which prevents microbial invasion. Thus, wound healing can be categorized into four stages which comprises of initial inflammatory phase, re-epithelialization, granulation tissue formation, and finally tissue remodeling [20]. This categorization is based upon histological examination or functional activities which are considerably overlapping. A deep interaction between cells and tissues involved in these phases finally results in wound healing [21].

Activated blood coagulation factors, complement components and damaged cells secrete growth factors and platelets which trigger chemotactic stimulus. Blood coagulation factors in conjunction with platelets initiate blood coagulation and activate fibrin. Fibronectin and vitronectin present in blood plasma form the substrate for cell migration involving keratinocytes. This is eventually followed by proteinases which result in scab formation around the wound [22]

As the blood coagulation process advances, within few hours neutrophils reach at the site of damaged tissue. They eliminate infective agents by phagocytizing them and promote blood coagulation and healing by secreting various factors [23]. Monocytes arrive at the wound within two days and differentiate into macrophages, to perform phagocytosis and antigen presenting functions. These macrophages regulate wound healing process by secreting, transforming growth factors-α and β, basic fibroblast growth factor, and platelet-derived growth factor [24]. Within few hours of inflammatory reaction, both re-epithelialization and granulation tissue formation takes place simultaneously. Keratinocytes present around the edges of the wound and in residues of skin appendages migrate into the wound and form a scab [25]. These keratinocytes are typically hyper-proliferative facilitating them to fill the damaged epithelial layer and reform the basement membrane within two days, restoring cellular contacts. This process leads to differentiation of keratinocytes into epidermal skin layer [26]. At almost the same time fibroblasts located around the undamaged dermis begin to proliferate and migrate as a result of the stimulus caused by the aforementioned growth factors, granulation tissue formation [27]. The extracellular around the wound is formed by proteoglycans, collagen type I and III, and collagen secreted by fibroblasts [22]. A portion of fibroblasts differentiate into myofibroblasts, which secrete actin, which builds up mechanical tension brings the edges of the wound closer resulting in wound contraction and finally wound closure [26]. The migration and proliferation of endothelial cells result in appearance of new blood vessels in granulation tissue [24]. The dermis remodeling phase of skin wound healing involves reduction of fibroblasts by apoptosis and removal of damaged blood vessels. The residual fibroblasts rearrange the collagen fiber, repeating collagen deposition and degradation for several months in order to recover the original tension of the skin [27].

Radicals produced by wounds are largely superoxide radical anions produced by neutrophils and macrophages, and also play an important role in removal of microorganisms and pathogens [28]. Superoxide radical anions are quickly transformed into hydrogen peroxide (H_2O_2) which is able to permeate microorganisms or pathogenic cell membranes by superoxide dismutase, promoting the formation of hypochlorous acid, chloramines, and aldehyde which are all maintained in more stable forms than H_2O_2, and are characterized by long half-lives. Thus, if H_2O_2 remain in the wound for extended period of time, acute inflammatory reactions can damage even normal cells [29].

Saponins present in various plant extracts possess extensive biological activities. They augment anti-oxidants and anti-inflammatory reactions. Saponins are one of several kinds of glycosides present in plants of high order [30]. Saponin types are named based upon their internal structure. A saponin referred to as fruticesaponin B is known to have a very high anti-inflammatory activity [31]. Navarro et al. [32] reported that anti-inflammatory activity of saponins is highly dependent on their chemical structure. In fact, both types of saponins tested in the study, prevented neutrophil access to wounds thereby decreasing chronic skin inflammatory reactions. On day 5, the wound healing rate was much faster in saponin-treated group than the control leading to complete joining of both sides of the incisional wounds on day 7. Except for day 1, during all time periods of evaluation, the wound area contracted more in the saponin-treated group than the control group. However, except day 1, the rate of keratin cell migration in the saponin-treated group was found to be higher than the control group during all periods. Another study reported that the burn wound area in a saponin-treated group was found to gradually increase up to day 4 then gradually decrease until day 20. In control group, the burn wound area gradually increased up to day 8 and then diminished in size [33]. The long lead time in healing the burn wound was due to inflammatory reaction around the burn wound which persisted longer [34]. Saponins were found to stimulate overexpression of factors, leading to proliferation of epidermal cells [35]. It was also found that rate of keratinocytes migration involved in re-epithelialization was faster in the saponin-treated group than in the control group. Hence, it was concluded that saponin not only enhances epidermal cell proliferation but also promotes migration of keratinocytes. The influx of inflammatory cells was measured in an animal wound model. On day 1 and day 3 it was found that the number of inflammatory cells in the saponin-treated group were much less in comparison to the control group. But were found to increase from day 5.

On day 7, the number of inflammatory cells were greater in the treated group than the control group. In burn wound number of leukocytes and macrophages increased up to day 9 [19]. Accumulation of macrophages was induced by IL-1β expression by hypoxia-inducible factor-1α. Hence, it is quite obvious that saponins are involved in inhibition of the inflammatory reaction at an early stage. Moreover, wound shrinkage increased sharply from day 3 onwards as compared to control group. Matrix remodeling analysis confirmed that matrix synthesis was promoted in the saponin-treated group compared to the control group. A recent study revealed that when saponin are used to treat skin tissue exposed to ultraviolet rays, collagen synthesis of fibroblasts was increased and expression of matrix metalloproteinases was inhibited [36]. It was also found that saponins increased collagen synthesis through phosphorylation of Smad 2 protein. Hence, saponins promote the regeneration of matrix at the wound site [37].

Hence, the literature findings very well indicate that saponins stimulates re-epithelialization of the wound and effectively inhibit early phase inflammatory reactions during and promotes matrix synthesis throughout the wound healing process. On the basis of the evidence existing in literature saponins are beneficial in healing incisional skin wounds. Ginseng leaves can be easily acquired and much cost effective compared to ginseng roots, hence there are several reports on isolation of active compounds from the Chinese ginseng leaves. These novel compounds were also tested for wound-healing activity [15].

3. Role of ginsenosides in wound healing

The principal active constituent of ginseng is a saponin called ginsenosides. Ginsenosides are found exclusively in the *Panax* species (ginseng); thus, they are also known as panaxosides. Nearly, 150 naturally occurring ginsenosides have been isolated from the roots, leaves, stems, fruits and flower heads of ginseng plant [38]. Ginsenosides are often divided into the Rb_1 group (characterized by the presence of protopanaxadiols: Rb_1, Rb_2, Rc and Rd) and the Rg_1 group (protopanaxatriols: Rg_1, Re, Rf and Rg_2). The remaining non-saponin components of ginseng are polysaccharides, polyacetylenes, peptides and amino acids. *P. ginseng* component, Rb_1 (G-Rb_1) has been studied extensively. It has been found to possess anti-inflammatory, antioxidant and antimicrobial activity. G-Rb_1 has also been found to enhance protein synthesis, neovascularization or angiogenesis and immunostimulation [39]. There have been inconsistent reports on effects of G-Rb_1 on dermal cell activities. This might be due to substantial variances in responses to G-Rb_1 in numerous cell lines being tested. An *in vitro* study revealed that G-Rb_1 had no cytotoxic effect on human keratinocyte (HaCaT) multiplication [19]. However, another study confirmed that G-Rb_1 improved the viability of human retinal pigment epithelial cells [40, 41]. An *in vivo* study showed that G-Rb_1 inhibits the chemoinvasion of endothelial cells during neovascularization [31]. However, another study showed that G-Rb_1 increases the number of blood vessels in burn wound areas of mice [42]. Schwann cell proliferation is significantly inhibited at 1 mg/ml, whereas 10 μg/ml of G-Rb_1 induces proliferation [40]. The effect of G-Rb1 on collagen synthesis is also uncertain. One study revealed that G-Rb_1 enhances collagen production in HaCaT cells [42]; however, G-Rb_1 reduced collagen levels in normal rat renal tubular epithelial cells (NRK-52E) [43]. Similarly, the effects of G-Rb_1 on cell function have been varied. Hence, the efficacy of G-Rb_1 on human dermal fibroblasts has not been confirmed. Lee et al. [44] treated cultured human dermal fibroblasts with one of six concentrations of *P. ginseng*: 0, 1, 10, 100 ng/ml and 1 and 10 μg/ml. Cell proliferation was determined 3 days post-treatment using the 3-(4,5-dimethylthiazol-2-yl)-2,5-diphenyl tetrazolium bromide assay. The collagen type I carboxy-terminal propeptide method was used to evaluate collagen synthesis. It was found that *P. ginseng* stimulated human dermal fibroblast proliferation and collagen synthesis at an optimal concentration of 10 ng/ml. This study, reported that G-Rb1 had significant positive effects on dermal fibroblast proliferation and collagen synthesis, which are essential factors during wound healing. *P. ginseng* generally is well tolerated. Although mild and reversible adverse effects of *P. ginseng* have been reported in cases where it was administered orally, including capsules, liquids or powders [45–49].

4. Summary and conclusion

Recently, the prime focus of wound specialists has been stimulation of wound healing. That is only possible when there is precise interplay of biological and molecular events, including cell migration, proliferation, extracellular matrix deposition and remodeling. The environment that favors the activities of key cell types need to be facilitated, clinically, for successful wound healing. These factors play a major role in regulating wound healing process by releasing various growth factors and cytokines. One such important cell type are fibroblasts. They perform numerous functions, including production of collagen, growth factors, antioxidants, initiating tissue remodeling, maintaining balanced levels of matrix-producing proteins and protease enzymes. A large number of clinical and experimental studies have confirmed that *P. ginseng* has multi-faceted effects in wound healing in humans, including angiogenesis, immunostimulation, and antimicrobial and anti-inflammatory actions. These activities contribute to wound healing potential of *P. ginseng* even in elderly population with greater predisposition to chronic wounds due to poor blood circulation, weak immune system, deficient nutritional factors and decreased cell activities. Hence ginseng is a potential candidate for incorporation in future dressings for wound management.

Author details

Dimple Sethi Chopra[1]*, Abhishek Gupta[2], Dhandeep Singh[1] and Nirmal Singh[1]

1 Department of Pharmaceutical Sciences and Drug Research, Punjabi University, Patiala, India

2 Institute of Health, Faculty of Education, Health and Wellbeing, University of Wolverhampton, Walsall, UK

*Address all correspondence to: dimplechopra@pbi.ac.in

IntechOpen

References

[1] Tinpun K, Nakpheng T, Padmavathi AR, Srichana T. *In vitro* studies of *Jatropha curcas* L. Latex spray formulation for wound healing applications. Turkish Journal of Pharmaceutical Sciences. 2020;**17**(3): 271-279. DOI: 10.4274/tjps.galenos.2019. 69875

[2] Guo S, DiPietro LA. Factors affecting wound healing. Journal of Dental Research. 2010;**89**(3):219-229

[3] Goldberg SR, Diegelmann RF. What makes wounds chronic. Surgical Clinics. 2020;**100**:681-693

[4] Ghosh PK, Gaba A. Phyto-extracts in wound healing. Journal of Pharmacy and Pharmaceutical Sciences. 2013; **16**(5):760-820

[5] Winter GD. Formation of the scab and the rate of epithelization of superficial wounds in the skin of the young domestic pig. Nature. 1962; **193**(4812):293-294

[6] Budovsky A, Yarmolinsky L, Ben-Shabat S. Effect of medicinal plants on wound healing. Wound Repair and Regeneration. 2015;**23**(2):171-183

[7] Zanzoni A, Montecchi-Palazzi L, Quondam MX. A molecular interaction database. FEBS Letters. 2002;**513**:135-140. DOI: 10.1016/s0014-5793(01) 03293-8

[8] Hsu S. Green tea and the skin. Journal of the American Academy of Dermatology. 2005;**52**:1049-1059

[9] Gupta A, Low WL, Radecka I, Britland ST, Amin MC, Martin C. Characterisation and in vitro antimicrobial activity of biosynthetic silver-loaded bacterial cellulose hydrogels. Journal of Microencapsulation. 2016;**33**(8):725-734

[10] Gupta A, Briffa SM, Swingler S, Gibson H, Kannapan V, Adamus G, et al. Synthesis of silver nanoparticles using curcumin-cyclodextrins loaded into bacterial cellulose based hydrogels for wound dressing applications. Biomacromolecules. 2020;**21**(5): 1802-1811

[11] Enoch S, Grey JE, Harding KG. Non-surgical and drug treatments. BMJ. 2006;**332**(7546):900-903. DOI: 10.1136/ bmj.332.7546.900

[12] Shedovea A, Leavesley D, Upton Z, Fan C. Wound healing and use of medicinal plants. Evidence-Based Complementary and Alternative Medicine. 2019;**2684108**:1-30

[13] Guimarães I, Baptista-Silva S, Pintado M, Oliveira AL. Polyphenols: A promising avenue in therapeutic solutions for wound care. Applied Sciences. 2021;**11**:1230-1250. DOI: 10.3390/app11031230

[14] Ghuman S, Ncube B, Finnie J, McGaw L, Njoya EM, Coopoosamy R, et al. Antioxidant, anti-inflammatory and wound healing properties of medicinal plant extracts used to treat wounds and dermatological disorders. South African Journal of Botany. 2019;**126**:232-240

[15] Wang ZY, Zhang J, Lu SL. Objective evaluation of burn and post-surgical scars and the accuracy of subjective scartype judgment. Chinese Medical Journal. 2008;**121**:2517-2520

[16] Sen CK, Khanna S, Gordillo G, Bagchi D, Bagchi M, Roy S. Oxygen, oxidants, and antioxidants in wound healing: An emerging paradigm. Annals of the New York Academy of Sciences. 2002;**957**:239-249

[17] Bishop A. Role of oxygen in wound healing. Journal of Wound Care. 2008;**17**:399-402

[18] Rodriguez PG, Felix FN, Woodley DT, Shim EK. The role of oxygen in wound healing: A review of the literature. Dermatologic Surgery. 2008;**34**:1159-1169

[19] Kimura Y, Sumiyoshi M, Kawahira K, Sakanaka M. Effects of ginseng saponins isolated from red ginseng roots on burn wound healing in mice. British Journal of Pharmacology. 2006;**148**:860-870

[20] Gonzalez ACDO, Costa TF, Andrade ZDA, Medrado ARAP. Wound healing—A literature review. Anais Brasileiros de Dermatologia. 2016;**91**: 614-620

[21] Toriseva M, Kahari VM. Proteinases in cutaneous wound healing. Cellular and Molecular Life Sciences. 2009; **66**:203-224

[22] Wang PH, Huang BS, Horng HC, Yeh CC, Chen YJ. Wound healing. Journal of the Chinese Medical Association. 2018;**81**:94-101

[23] Eming SA, Krieg T, Davidson JM. Inflammation in wound repair: Molecular and cellular mechanisms. The Journal of Investigative Dermatology. 2007;**127**:514-525

[24] Janis JE, Harrison B. Wound healing: Part I. Basic science. Plastic and Reconstructive Surgery. 2014; **133**:199e-207e

[25] Patel S, Srivastava S, Singh MR, Singh D. Mechanistic insight into diabetic wounds: Pathogenesis, molecular targets and treatment strategies to pace wound healing. Biomedicine and Pharmacotherapy. 2019;**112**:108615

[26] Tottoli EM, Dorati R, Genta I, Chiesa E, Pisani S, Conti B. Skin wound healing process and new emerging technologies for skin wound care and

regeneration. Pharmaceutics. 2020; **12**:735

[27] Akasaka Y, Ono I, Kamiya T, et al. The mechanisms underlying fibroblast apoptosis regulated by growth factors during wound healing. Journal of Pathology. 2010;**221**(3):285-299

[28] Eming SA, Martin P, Tomic-Canic M. Wound repair and regeneration: Mechanisms, signaling, and translation. Science Translational Medicine. 2014;**265**:265sr6

[29] Kasuya A, Tokura Y. Attempts to accelerate wound healing. Journal of Dermatological Science. 2014;**76**(3):169-172

[30] Wu QB, Wang Y, Liang L, Jiang Q, Guo ML, Zhang JJ. Novel triterpenoid saponins from the seeds of *Celosia argentea* L. Natural Product Research. 2013;**27**(15):1353-1360

[31] Ashour ML, Youssef FS, Gad HA, El-Readi MZ, Bouzabata A, Abuzeid RM, et al. Evidence for the anti-inflammatory activity of *Bupleurum marginatum* (*Apiaceae*) extracts using *in vitro* and *in vivo* experiments supported by virtual screening. Journal of Pharmacy and Pharmacology. 2018;**70**(7):952-963. DOI: 10.1111/jphp.12904

[32] Navarro P, Giner RM, Recio MC, Manez S, Cerda-Nicolas M, Ríos JL. *In vivo* anti-inflammatory activity of saponins from *Bupleurum rotundifolium*. Life Sciences. 2001;**68**:1199-1206

[33] Kovacs EJ, Grabowski KA, Duffner LA, Plackett TP, Gregory MS. Survival and cell mediated immunity after burn injury in aged mice. Journal of the American Aging Association. 2002;**25**(1):3-9. DOI: 10.1007/s11357-002-0001-4

[34] Madaghiele M, Demitri C, Sannino A, Ambrosio L. Polymeric

hydrogels for burn wound care: Advanced skin wound dressings and regenerative templates. Burns Trauma. 2014;**2**(4):153-161. DOI: 10.4103/2321-3868.143616

[35] Choi S. Epidermis proliferative effect of the *Panax ginseng* ginsenoside Rb2. Archives of Pharmacal Research. 2002;**25**:71-76

[36] Kim YG, Sumiyoshi M, Sakanaka M, Kimura Y. Effects of ginseng saponins isolated from red ginseng on ultraviolet B-induced skin aging in hairless mice. European Journal of Pharmacology. 2009;**602**:148-156

[37] Lee J, Jung E, Lee J, Huh S, Kim J, Park M, et al. *Panax ginseng* induces human type I collagen synthesis through activation of Smad signaling. Journal of Ethnopharmacology. 2007;**109**:29-34

[38] Hong CE, Lyu SY. Anti-inflammatory and anti-oxidative effects of Korean red ginseng extract in human keratinocytes. Immune Network. 2011;**11**:42-49

[39] Yang N, Chen P, Tao Z, Zhou N, Gong X, Xu Z, et al. Beneficial effects of ginsenoside-Rg1 on ischemia-induced angiogenesis in diabetic mice. Acta Biochimica et Biophysica Sinica. 2012;**44**:999-1005

[40] Cho JS, Moon YM, Um JY, Moon JH, Park IH, Lee HM. Inhibitory effect of ginsenoside Rg1 on extracellular matrix production via extracellular signal-regulated protein kinase/activator protein 1 pathway in nasal polyp-derived fibroblasts. Experimental Biology and Medicine. 2012;**237**:663-669

[41] Wu HT, Chen XX, Xiong LJ. Experimental study of proliferation of Schwann cells cultured with ginsenoside Rb1. Zhongguo Xiu Fu Chong Jian Wai Ke Za Zhi. 2003;**17**:26-29

[42] Kim YS, Cho IH, Jeong MJ, Jeong SJ, Nah SY, Cho YS, et al. Therapeutic effect of total ginseng saponin on skin wound healing. Journal of Ginseng Research. 2011;**35**(3):360-367

[43] Xie XS, Liu HC, Fan JM, Li HJ. Effects of ginsenoside Rb1 on TGF-beta1 induced p47phox expression and extracellular matrix accumulation in rat renal tubular epithelial cells. Sichuan Da Xue Xue Ba Yi Xue Ban. 2009;**40**:106-110

[44] Lee GY, Park KG, Namgoong S, Han SK, Jeong SH, Dhong ES, et al. Effects of *Panax ginseng* extract on human dermal fibroblast proliferation and collagen synthesis. International Wound Journal. 2016;**13**(suppl. s1):42-46

[45] Shergis JL, ZhangAL ZW, Xue CC. *Panax ginseng* in randomised controlled trials: A systematic review. Phytotherapy Research. 2013;**27**:949-965

[46] Coon JT, Ernst E. *Panax ginseng*: A systematic review of adverse effects and drug interactions. Drug Safety. 2002;**25**:323-344

[47] Kim WK, Song SY, Oh WK, Kaewsuwan S, Tran TL, Kim WS, et al. Wound-healing effect of ginsenoside Rd from leaves of *Panax ginseng* via cyclic AMP-dependent protein kinase pathway. European Journal of Pharmacology. 2013;**12**:1-9. DOI: 10.1016/j.ejphar.2013.01.048i

[48] Park S, Daily JW, Lee J. Can topical use of ginseng or ginsenosides accelerate wound healing? Journal of Medicinal Food. 2016;**21**(11):1075-1076

[49] Sengupta S, Toh SA, Sellers LA, Skepper JN, Koolwijk P, Leung HW, et al. Modulating angiogenesis: The yin and the yang in ginseng. Circulation. 2004;**110**:1219-1225

Chapter 5

Bioinformatics Exploration of Ginseng: A Review

Toluwase Hezekiah Fatoki

Abstract

Ginseng contains an extraordinarily complex mixture of chemical constituents that can vary with the species used, the place of origin, and the growing conditions. Various computational analyses which include genomics, transcriptomics, proteomics and bioinformatics have been used to study ginseng plant. A genome-scale metabolic network offers a holistic view of ginsenoside biosynthesis, helps to predict genes associated with the production of pharmacologically vital dammarane-type ginsenosides, and provides insight for improving medicinal values of ginseng by genomics-based breeding. The draft genomic architecture of tetraploid *P. ginseng* cultivar (cv.) Chunpoong (ChP) by de novo genome assembly, was found to be 2.98 Gbp and consist of 59,352 annotated genes. Presently, bioinformatics exploration of ginseng includes studies on its P-glycoproteins, the impact of cytochrome P-450 on ginseng pharmacokinetics, as well as target prediction and differential gene expression network analyses. This study applauded Betasitosterol and Daucosterin as ginseng bioactive constituents that have several potential pharmacological effects in human, by modulating several proteins which include androgen receptor, HMG-CoA reductase, interlukin-2, and consequently impact the signaling cascade of several kinases such as mitogen-activated protein kinases (MAPKs), as well as many transcription factors such as polycomb protein SUZ12.

Keywords: Ginseng, bioinformatics, transcriptomics, genomics, bioactive, pharmacokinetics

1. Introduction

Ginseng is a slow-growing, deciduous, perennial plant of the *Araliaceae* family which includes *Panax ginseng* (*Renshen*, Chinese or Korean ginseng), *Panax japonicus* (Japanese ginseng) and *Panax quinquefolius* (*Xiyangshen*, American ginseng) among others [1]. Ginseng contains an extraordinarily complex mixture of chemical constituents that can vary with the species used, the place of origin, and the growing conditions [2]. Ginsengs has found therapeutic application such as anti-inflammatory, anti-haemostatic, antioxidant, anticancer, anti-diabetic, antiaging, anti-depressive, immunomodulatory, analgesic, neuroprotection, memory and learning enhancement effects in animals and humans [1, 3–7]. Various computational analyses which include genomics, transcriptomics, proteomics and bioinformatics have been used to study ginseng plant [4, 8–10].

1.1 Ginseng genomics and biosynthesis of ginsenosides

A genome-scale metabolic network offers a holistic view of ginsenoside biosynthesis, helps to predict genes associated with the production of pharmacologically vital dammarane-type ginsenosides, and provides insight for improving medicinal values of ginseng by genomics-based breeding [11]. The draft genomic architecture of tetraploid *P. ginseng* cultivar (cv.) Chunpoong, by de novo genome assembly, was reported to be 2.98 Gbp and consist of 59,352 annotated genes [11]. Recently, a dynamic database was built that integrates a draft genome sequence, transcriptome profiles, and annotation datasets of ginseng, which is publicly available (http://ginsengdb.snu.ac.kr/) for the use of scientific community around the globe for exploring the valuable resources for a range of research fields related to *P. ginseng* and few other species [4]. Transcriptome analysis has identified 100 *Panax ginseng* cytochrome P450 (*PgCYP*) genes, whose expressions were significantly correlated with variation of nine mono- and total-ginsenoside contents, while further association study identified five SNPs and three InDels from six *PgCYP* genes that were significantly associated with the ginsenoside contents in the four-year-old roots of 42 genotypes [9].

2. Ginsenosides: structure, pharmacokinetics and mechanism

Ginsenosides are specific types of triterpene saponin, a broad group of chemical compounds. Ginsenosides are found nearly exclusively in Panax species (ginseng) and up to now more than 150 naturally occurring ginsenosides have been isolated from different organs of ginseng [12]. Ginsenosides appear to be responsible for most of the activities of ginseng including anti-diabetic, anti-allergic, anticarcinogenic, anti-inflammatory, anti-atherosclerotic, antihypertensive, and immuno-modulatory effects as well as anti-stress activity and effects on the central nervous system [6]. The structures of ginsenosides Rb1 and Rg1 are shown in **Figure 1**.

2.1 Structure of ginsenosides

Shi *et al.* [13] have reported that the seven major ginsenosides (Rg1, Re, Rb1, Rc, Rb2, Rb3 and Rd) were present in various parts of Chinese ginseng of various ages. Ginsenoside content is higher in the leaf and root hair but lower in the stem than that in other parts of the plant and that the total content of ginsenosides in the leaf decreases with age [1, 13]. Ginsenosides are divided into three main categories, the 20(S)-protopanaxadiol, 20(S)-proto- panaxatriol and oleanane families according

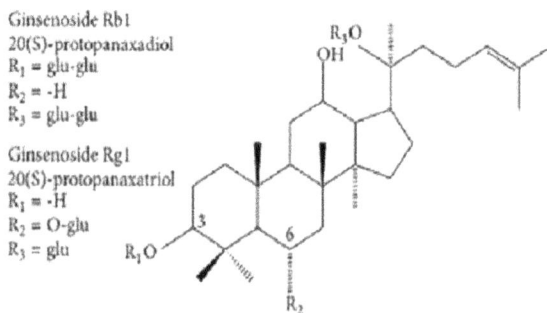

Figure 1.
Structures of ginsenosides Rb1 and Rg1. (Adapted from [5]).

to the number and position of sugar moieties on the sterol chemical structure. it is difficult to clarify the influence of the sugar moiety at different positions on pharmacological actions [14].

2.2 ADME of ginsenosides

Absorption, distribution, metabolism and excretion (ADME) describe the pharmacokinetics and pharmacodynamics of a single or more compounds in an organism such as human, mouse etc. The knowledge of pharmacokinetics of ginsenoside and its metabolites is very imperative in designing an optimal dosage regimen and minimizing the adverse effect that may result from ginseng-drugs interaction. The polar ginsenosides include Rg1, Re, Rb1, Rc, Rb2, Rb3, and Rd., while less polar ginsenosides include Rg2, Rg3, Rg5, Rh2, Rk1, and Rs4 [15, 16]. Protopanaxadiol ginsenosides are metabolized to ginsenoside compound K by the intestinal microflora in humans. Ginsenoside compound K (20-O-β-D-glucopyranosyl-20(S)-protopanaxadiol), is found in the blood stream of humans as an active metabolite after oral administration of protopanaxadiol ginsenosides Rb1, Rb2, Rc, and Rd., and has significantly higher mean maximum plasma concentration and significantly lower half-life when compare to the ginsenoside Rb1 [17].

According to Qi et al., [18], the ginseng saponins have low absorption rate and characterized by extensive metabolism in the gastrointestinal tract, poor membrane permeability, and low solubility of deglycosylated products; and with less than 5% dose bioavailability of the protopanaxadiol (PPD) group of saponins (ginsenosides Ra3, Rb1, Rd., Rg3, and Rh2) and of the protopanaxatriol (PPT) group of saponins (ginsenosides Rg1, Re, Rh1, and R1) were less than 5%. However, PPT saponins have better bioavailability than PPD saponins, which may be due to the fact that PPD saponins degrade faster than PPT saponins. Study on ginseng absorption by HPLC analysis, showed that Rb1 (4.35%) and Rg1 (18.40%) were absorbed, respectively [19].

Study on the effect of American ginseng and Asian ginseng extracts on gene expression of the hepatic cytochrome P450 enzyme in elderly humans, has shown that protopanaxadiol (PPD), protopanaxatriol (PPT) and their metabolites, moderately inhibited CYP2C9 activity and strongly inhibited CYP3A4 activity [20, 21]. Henderson et al., [22] have studied the effects of seven naturally occurring ginsenosides Rb1, Rb2, Rc, Rd., Re, Rf, and Rg1 and eleutherosides B and

S.No	Constituents	References
1.	Ginsenine	[24]
2	betasitosterol, 20(R)-protopanaxatriol, daucosterin, 20(R)-ginsenoside-Rg3	[25]
3	isoginsenoside-Rh(3), ginsenoside-Rb(1), -Rb(2), −Rc, −Rd, -Re, − Rg(1), -Rh(1), -Rh(2).	[26]
4	Daucosterin; 20(R)-dammarane-3beta,12beta,20,25-tetrol (25-OHPPD); 20(R)-dammarane-3beta,6alpha,12beta,20,25-pentol (25-OH-PPT); 20(S)-protopanaxadiol (PPD); 20(S)-ginsenoside-Rh(2) (Rh2); 20(S)-ginsenoside-Rg(3) (Rg3); 20(S)-ginsenoside-Rg(2) (Rg2); 20(S)-ginsenoside-Rg(1) (Rg1); 20(S)-ginsenoside-Rd (Rd); 20(S)-ginsenoside-Re (Re); 20(S)-ginsenoside-Rb(1) (Rb1).	[27]
5	Panaxadione, ginsenosides Rd., Re, and Rg2	[28]

Table 1.
Chemical constituents of P. ginseng.

S.No	Ginsenoside	Mechanism	Reference
1	Rb1	protects hippocampal neuron, enhance insulin/IGF-1 signaling, inhibited GSK-3β-mediated C/EBP homologous protein (CHOP) signaling	[29–32]
2	Rb$_2$	Down-regulation of matrix metalloproteinase (MMP)-2	[33]
3	Rg1	Downregulation of nuclear factor-kappa B (NF-κB)/nitric oxide (NO) signaling pathway, increases the expression of insulin growth factor I receptor (IGF-IR)	[34–35]
4	Rd	Phosphoinositide-3-kinase/AKT and phosphoextracellular signal-regulated protein kinase (ERK) 1/2 pathways, suppress poly(ADP-ribose) polymerase-1, protein tyrosine kinase activation, the upregulation of the endogenous antioxidant system and GAP-43 expression	[5, 36, 37]
5	Re	PREVENT the reduction of H(+)-ATPase activity	[38]
6	Rg3	Modulation of three modules of MAP kinases, P-gp (P-glycoprotein) inhibition, modulation of Ephrin receptor pathway, inhibits NMDA receptor by increasing the concentration of glycine, suppression of TPA-induced cyclooxygenase-2 (COX-2) expression	[39–42]

Table 2.
The molecular mechanism of ginsenosides pharmacological activities.

E (active components of the ginseng root) on the catalytic activity of *c*DNA expressed CYPs (CYP1A2, CYP2C9, CYP2C19, CYP2D6 and CYP3A4) in *in vitro* experiments. They found that the ginsenosides and eleutherosides tested are not likely to inhibit the metabolism of co-administered medications in which the primary route of elimination is via cytochrome P450 [22]. Comprehensive review of the ginseng active compounds pharmacokinetics, drug–drug interaction, and influence of cytochrome P450 has been published [23]. Chemical constituents of *P. ginseng* and mechanisms of selected ginseng compounds are shown in **Tables 1** and **2** respectively.

3. Bioinformatics analyses of ginsenosides

A study has proposed a novel method to explore underlying mechanisms of multiple actions of multiple constituents of Ginseng (*Panax ginseng*) against cancers, and the bioinformatics analyses was initiated with proteins regulated by ginsenoside rb1/re/rg1, using standard tools such as ChEMBL, STRING, DAVID and KEGG [43].

In the study conducted by Yan et al. [44] to identify immunomodulatory bio-markers in an immune cell induced by ginseng, microarray assays were carried out to identify differentially expressed genes associated with American ginseng (*Panax quinquefolius*) exposure to 4 groups of Murine splenic cells from adult male C57BL/6 (B6) mice which were isolated to mimic 4 basic pathophysiological states. The microarray data obtained was analyzed with Partek Genomics Suite software while DAVID Bioinformatics Resources 6.7 was used for functional annotation clustering. The effect of American ginseng on the interferon gamma signaling functions was obtained by the use of Interferome software [44].

In their study, Zhu et al. [8], have reported two major *Panax ginseng* glycoprotein (PGG-1 and PGG-2) obtained by high performance liquid chromatography, with the molecular weights of 1.5 KDa and 8.2 KDa respectively calculated by gel permeation chromatography. The ginseng samples were analyzed by LC–MS using a nano-flow RP-HPLC online-coupled to a Q Exactive mass spectrophotometer operating in the positive ion mode. The raw MS files were analyzed and searched against the UniProt ginseng protein sequence database using Byonic software (Version 2.3.5). The computed parameters of PGG determined by MS include theoretical isoelectric point (pI), instability index, aliphatic index and grand average of hydropathicity (GRAVY). The aliphatic index of PGG-1 ranged from 0 to 130, with an average of 48.23; the aliphatic index of PGG-2 ranged from 61.25 to 195.71, with an average of 129.41 [8].

Bioinformatics network analysis has been used to analyzed a combination of ginseng and arginine regimen, ginseng and lingzhi as well as ginseng and gingko regimens [45, 46], in order to understand potential impact of drug–drug interaction (agonism or antagonism) based on common pathways.

3.1 *In silico* target prediction and gene expression network of key ginseng constituents

The ligands (Ginsenoside Rb1, Rc, Rg3, Re, F1, C; Betasitosterol, Panaxadione, Daucosterin (also known as Sitogluside or Eleutheroside A), and 20(R)-protopanaxatriol) were subjected to *in silico* target prediction on Swiss TargetPrediction server where *Homo sapiens* was selected as target organism [47] as shown in **Table 3**. Forty-five (45) genes (PTAFR, IL2, STAT3, VEGFA, FGF1, FGF2, HPSE, PSEN1, PSENEN, NCSTN, BCL2L1, PRKCA, HSD11B1, CYP19A1, SIRT2, PTPN1, CCR1, VDR, PTPN11, NR1I2, REN, BACE1, NR3C1, INSR, ITK,

S.No	Constituents	Target Genes	% probability	Possible effect
1	Ginsenoside Rb1, Rg3, Rc, Re, F1, C,	PTAFR, IL2, STAT3, VEGFA, FGF1, FGF2, HPSE, PSEN1, PSENEN, NCSTN, BCL2L1	10	Immunomodulatory, anti-haemostatic, anti-cancer
2	Panaxadione	PRKCA, HSD11B1, CYP19A1, SIRT2, PTPN1, CCR1, VDR, PTPN11, NR1I2, REN, BACE1, NR3C1, INSR, ITK, F2R	20	Anti-inflammatory, anti-diabetic
3	Betasitosterol	AR, HMGCR, CYP51A1, NPC1L1, NR1H3, CYP19A1, CYP17A1, RORC, ESR1, ESR2	35–70	Anti-depressive, neuroprotection, anti-cancer
4	Daucosterin	STAT3, IL2	20–60	Immunomodulatory, anti-cancer, anti-inflammatory
5	20(R)-protopanaxatriol	PTPN1, CYP2C19, CHRM2, SLC6A2, SLC6A4, AR, ACHE, HSD11B1, ESR1, CYP19A1, ATP12A, NR1H3, HMGCR, CYP51A1, NPC1L1	20	Anti-depressive, anti-hypertension

Table 3.
Predicted genes of selected Ginseng constituent.

F2R, AR, HMGCR, CYP51A1, NPC1L1, NR1H3, CYP19A1, CYP17A1, RORC, ESR1, ESR2, CYP2C19, CHRM2, SLC6A2, SLC6A4, ACHE, HSD11B1, ATP12A, HMGCR, CYP51A1) were extracted from the predicted targets and subjected to expression network analyses (transcription factor enrichment analysis, protein–protein interaction network expansion and kinase enrichment analysis), using eXpression2Kinases (X2K) Web server [48] as shown **Figures 2–5**.

The genes that were targeted by Betasitosterol (**Table 3**) have greater than 30% probability (35–70%), Daucosterin targeted Interleukin-2 (IL2) with 60% probability, while others were less than 30%. The best target of Betasitosterol is Androgen Receptor (AR), followed by 3-hydroxy-3-methylglutaryl-coenzyme A (HMG-CoA) reductase, Cytochrome P450 51, Niemann-Pick C1-like protein 1, LXR-alpha, Cytochrome P450 19A1, Cytochrome P450 17A1, Nuclear receptor ROR-gamma and others.

This study shows that SUZ12 has the highest score as transcription factor influenced by the ginseng, this is followed by STAT3, RUNX1, FOS, VDR, RCOR1,

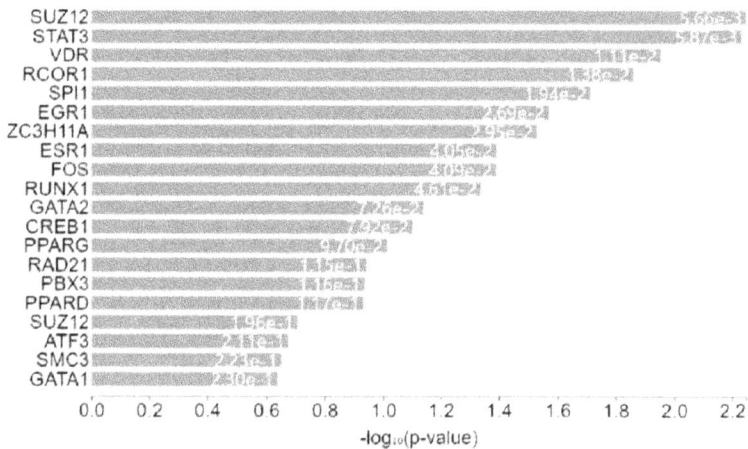

Figure 2.
Transcription Factor Enrichment Analysis (TFEA).

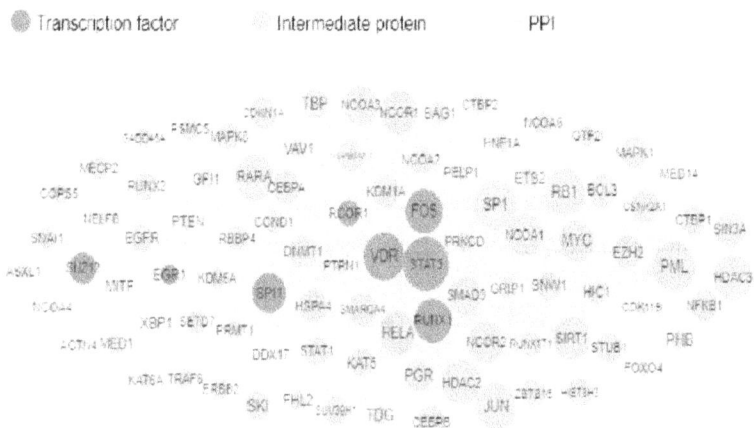

Figure 3.
Protein–Protein Interaction.

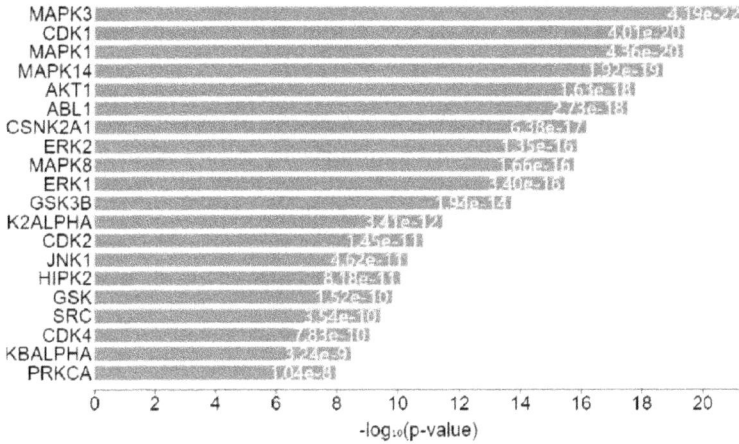

Figure 4.
Kinase Enrichment Analysis (KEA).

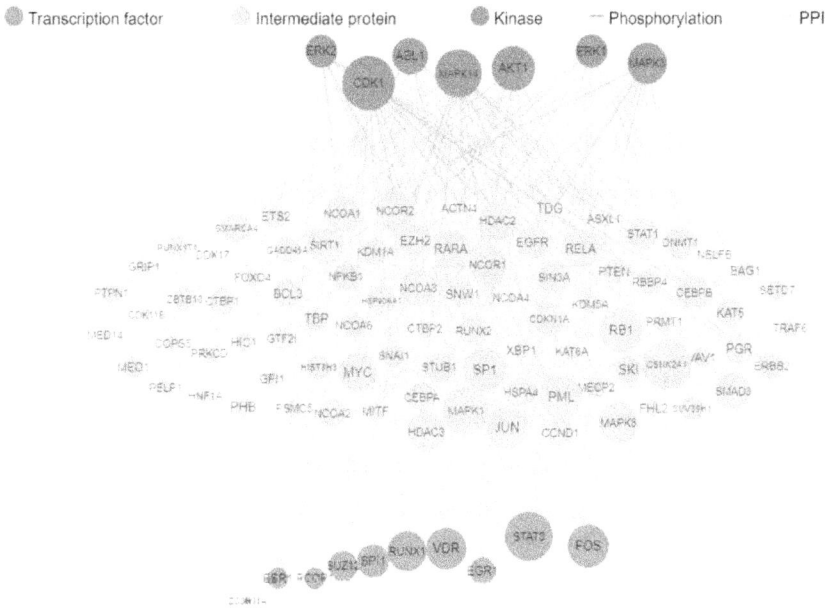

Figure 5.
eXpression2Kinases Network.

SPI1 and EGR1 (**Figures 2** and **3**). The kinases that were impacted by the action of ginseng active constituents include MAPK1, MAPK14, AKT1, CDK1, ABL1, ERK1 and ERK2 (**Figure 4**). Moreover, major intermediate proteins JUN, RARA, NCOR1, MYC, RB1, HDAC2, CSNK2A1 and others (**Figure 5**).

Zhang et al. [49] have reported ginsenoside, stigmasterol, β-sterol, β-elemene and β-selinene, kaempferol, panaxynol, ginsenoyne A, fumarine, girinimbin, elemicin, dauricine, and maltol, as part of secondary metabolites produced by ginseng. However, network analysis of ginseng-associated targets ginseng in treatment of depression which could occur in post-COVID19 period, identified AKT1, CASP3,

NOS3, TNF, and PPARG as the core genes in protein–protein interaction network, and that ginsenoside Re, ginsenoside Rg1, frutinone A and kaempferol were the key ingredients in ginseng for immune-regulation [50].

Based on curated data on UniProt database (www.uniprot.org), androgen receptor (Uniprot ID: P10275) involves in positive regulation of MAPK cascade, NF-kappaB transcription factor activity, insulin-like growth factor receptor signaling pathway, and transcription by RNA polymerase II and III, as well as negative regulation of transcription by RNA polymerase II, epithelial cell proliferation, and extrinsic apoptotic signaling pathway. HMG-CoA reductase (UniProt ID: P04035) involves in positive regulation of ERK1 and ERK2 cascade, stress-activated MAPK cascade, cardiac muscle cell apoptotic process, smooth muscle cell proliferation, and cholesterol homeostasis, as well as negative regulation of MAP kinase activity, wound healing, and striated muscle cell apoptotic process, and it also give response to ethanol. Interleukin-2 (UniProt ID: P60568) involves in positive regulation of inflammatory response, transcription by RNA polymerase II, tyrosine phosphorylation of STAT protein, interferon-gamma production, B cell and activated T cell proliferation and immunoglobulin secretion, as well as negative regulation of inflammatory response, heart contraction, B cell apoptotic process, and lymphocyte proliferation, and it also give response to ethanol.

A comprehensive review of betasitosterol has reported several therapeutic potentials which include antioxidant, antipyretic, anti-inflammatory, anti-arthritic, and antimicrobial activities, as well as anti-cancer, anti-diabetic, antihyperlipidemic, anti-atherosclerosis, anti-pulmonary tuberculosis, angiogenic, immune modulation and anti-HIV effects [51].

4. Conclusion

Knowledge of bioinformatics has not been fully applied to the study of ginseng in proportionality to the acclaimed medicinal properties from the ethnobotanical use.

This study has applauded Betasitosterol and Daucosterin as ginseng bioactive constituents that have several potential pharmacological effects in human, by modulating several proteins which include androgen receptor, HMG-CoA reductase, interlukin-2, and consequently impact the signaling cascade of several kinases such as Mitogen-activated protein kinases (MAPKs), as well as many transcription factors such as Polycomb protein SUZ12. Moreover, difference in pharmacological outcome of aqueous ginseng extract and ethanolic ginseng extract would necessitate holistic approach of extraction. Furthermore, chemical biology and *in silico* simulation of pharmacological potential of ginseng bioactive compounds (such as molecular docking and dynamics, drug–drug interaction) will yield significant insights to the presently unexplored molecular mechanisms of action to explain the therapeutic effect of ginseng.

Acknowledgements

This research has no acknowledgment.

Conflict of interest

The authors declare no conflict of interest.

Author details

Toluwase Hezekiah Fatoki
Department of Biochemistry, Federal University Oye, Oye-Ekiti, Ekiti State, Nigeria

*Address all correspondence to: toluwase.fatoki@fuoye.edu.ng;
hezekiahfatoki@gmail.com

IntechOpen

References

[1] Wang H., Peng D., and Xie J., Ginseng leaf-stem: bioactive constituents and pharmacological functions. Chinese Medicine 2009, 4:20. DOI:10.1186/1749-8546-4-20

[2] Lee SY, Kim YK, Park N-II, Kim CS, Lee CY, and Park SU. Chemical constituents and biological activities of the berry of *Panax ginseng*. Journal of Medicinal Plants Research 2010, 4(5), 349-353. https://academicjournals.org/journal/JMPR/article-full-text-pdf/8FAA32115670/

[3] Shi Z-Y, Zeng J-Z., and Wong A.S.T. Chemical Structures and Pharmacological Profiles of Ginseng Saponins. Molecules 2019, *24*, 2443; DOI:10.3390/molecules24132443

[4] Jayakodi M., Choi B-S., Lee S-C., Kim N-H., Park J.Y. et al., Ginseng Genome Database: an open-access platform for genomics of *Panax ginseng*. BMC Plant Biology (2018) 18:62. DOI: 10.1186/s12870-018-1282-9

[5] Rokot NT, Kairupan TS, Cheng K-C, Runtuwene J., Kapantow NH., Amitani M., Morinaga A, Amitani H., Asakawa A., and Inui A., (2016). A Role of Ginseng and Its Constituents in the Treatment of Central Nervous System Disorders. Evidence-Based Complementary and Alternative Medicine, Volume 2016, Article ID 2614742, 1-7. DOI:10.1155/2016/2614742

[6] Lu JM, Yao Q, Chen C (2009). Ginseng compounds: an update on their molecular mechanisms and medical applications. Curr. Vasc. Pharmacol. 7: 293-302. DOI: 10.2174/157016109788340767

[7] Xie JT, Mchendale S, Yuan CS (2005). Ginseng and diabetes. Am. J. Chin. Med. 33: 397-404. DOI: 10.1142/S0192415X05003004

[8] Zhu D., Fang X., Chen Y., et al., Structure-activity relationship analysis of Panax ginseng glycoproteins with cytoprotective effects using LC-MS/MS and bioinformatics, International Journal of Biological Macromolecules (2020), DOI: 10.1016/j.ijbiomac.2020.05.034

[9] Zhao M., Lin Y., Wang Y., Li X., Han Y., Wang K., Sun C., Wang Y., and Zhang M., (2019). Transcriptome analysis identifies strong candidate genes for ginsenoside biosynthesis and reveals its underlying molecular mechanism in *Panax ginseng* C.A. Meyer. 9:615, 1-10. DOI:10.1038/s41598-018-36349-5

[10] Xu J, Chu Y, Liao B, Xiao S, Yin Q, Bai R, Su H, et al., (2017). *Panax ginseng* genome examination for ginsenoside biosynthesis. GigaScience, 6, 2017, 1-15. DOI: 10.1093/gigascience/gix093

[11] Kim N-H, Jayakodi M, Lee S-C, Choi B-S, Jang W, Lee J, et al., (2018). Genome and evolution of the shade-requiring medicinal herb *Panax ginseng*. Plant Biotechnology Journal (2018) 16, 1904-1917. DOI: 10.1111/pbi.12926

[12] Christensen LP. Ginsenosides chemistry, biosynthesis, analysis, and potential health effects. Adv Food Nutr Res. 2009;55:1-99. DOI: 10.1016/S1043-4526(08)00401-4.

[13] Shi W, Wang Y, Li J, Zhang H, Ding L: Investigation of ginsenosides in different parts and ages of Panax ginseng. Food Chemistry 2007, 102:664-668. DOI: 10.1016/j.foodchem.2006.05.053

[14] Liu Z-Q. Chemical Insights into Ginseng as a Resource for Natural Antioxidants. Chem. Rev. 2012, 112, 3329-3355. DOI:10.1021/cr100174k.

[15] Lau AJ, Seo BH, Woo SO, Koh HL. High-performance liquid chromatographic method with quantitative comparisons of whole chromatograms of raw and steamed Panax notoginseng. J Chromatogr A. 2004,1057:141-149. DOI: 10.1016/j. chroma.2004.09.069

[16] Kwon SW, Han SB, Park IH, Kim JM, Park MK, Park JH. Liquid chromatographic determination of less polar ginsenosides in processed ginseng. J Chromatogr A. 2001;921:335-339. DOI: 10.1016/s0021-9673(01)00869-x

[17] Kim H-K, Pharmacokinetics of ginsenoside Rb1 and its metabolite compound K after oral administration of Korean Red Ginseng extract. J Ginseng Res 2013; 37(4): 451-456. DOI: 10.5142/jgr.2013.37.451

[18] Qi LW, Wang CZ, Du GJ, Zhang ZY, Calway T, Yuan CS. Metabolism of ginseng and its interactions with drugs. Curr Drug Metab. 2011;12(9):818-822. DOI: 10.2174/138920011797470128.

[19] Xu QF, Fang XL, Chen DF. Pharmacokinetics and bioavailability of ginsenoside Rb1 and Rg1 from *Panax notoginseng* in rats. Journal of Ethnopharmacol. 2003; 84: 187-192. DOI: 10.1016/s0378-8741(02)00317-3

[20] Gurley BJ, Gardner SF, Hubbard MA, Williams DK, Gentry WB, Cui YY, Ang CYW. Clinical assessment of effects of botanical supplementation on cytochrome P450 phenotypes in the elderly - St John's wort, garlic oil, *Panax ginseng* and *Ginkgo biloba*. Drug Aging. 2005; 22(6):525-539. DOI: 10.2165/00002512-200522060-00006

[21] Liu Y, Zhang JW, Li W, Ma H, Sun J, Deng MC, Yang L. Ginsenoside metabolites, rather than naturally occurring ginsenosides, lead to inhibition of human cytochrome P450

enzymes. Toxicol. Sci. 2006; 91(2):356-364. DOI: 10.1093/toxsci/kfj164

[22] Henderson GL, Harkey MR, Gershwin ME, Hackman RM, Stern JS, Stresser DM. Effects of ginseng components on c-DNA-expressed cytochrome P450 enzyme catalytic activity. Life Sci 1999; 65(15):PL209–PL214. DOI: 10.1016/s0024-3205(99)00407-5

[23] Yang L., Liu Y., and Liu C-X., Metabolism and pharmacokinetics of ginsenosides. Asian Journal of Pharmacodynamics and Pharmacokinetics 2006; 6(2):103-120.

[24] Wang JY, Li XG, Yang XW. Ginsenine, a new alkaloid from the berry of *Panax ginseng* C. A. Meyer. J. Asian Nat. Prod. Res. 2006;8: 605-608. DOI: 10.1080/10286020500208444

[25] Zhao YQ, Yuan CL. Chemical constituents of the fruit of *Panax ginseng* C. A. Meyer. Zhongguo Zhong Yao Za Zhi. 1993;18: 296-297.

[26] Wang JY, Li XG, Zheng YN, Yang XW. Isoginsenoside-Rh3, a new triterpenoid saponin from the fruits of *Panax ginseng* C. A. Mey. J. Asian Nat. Prod. Res. 2004;6: 289-293. DOI: 10.1080/10286020310001595980

[27] Wang W, Zhao Y, Rayburn E, Hill D, Wang H, Zhang R. *In vitro* anti-cancer activity and structure–activity relationships of natural products isolated from fruits of *Panax ginseng*. Cancer Chemother. Pharmacol. 2007;59: 589-601. DOI: 10.1007/s00280-006-0300-z

[28] Sugimoto S, Nakamura S, Matsuda H, Kitagawa N, Yoshikawa M. Chemical Constituents from Seeds of *Panax ginseng*: Structure of New Dammarane-Type Triterpene Ketone, Panaxadione, and HPLC Comparisons of Seeds and Flesh. Chem. Pharm.

Bull. 2009;57: 283-287. DOI: 10.1248/cpb.57.283

[29] Attele A.S., Wu J.A., and Yuan C.S. Ginseng pharmacology: multiple constituents and multiple actions. Biochemical Pharmacology. 1999;581(11),1685-1693. DOI: 10.1016/s0006-2952(99)00212-9

[30] Shang W, Yang Y, Zhou L, Jiang B, Jin H, Chen M. Ginsenoside Rb1 stimulates glucose uptake through insulin-like signaling pathway in 3T3-L1 adipocytes. J Endocrinol 2008; 198:561-569. DOI: 10.1677/JOE-08-0104

[31] Park S, Ahn IS, Kwon DY, Ko BS, Jun WK. Ginsenosides Rb1 and Rg1 suppress triglyceride accumulation in 3T3-L1 adipocytes and enhance beta-cell insulin secretion and viability in Min6 cells via PKA-dependent pathways. Biosci Biotechnol Biochem 2008; 72:2815-2823. DOI: 10.1271/bbb.80205

[32] Liu, D.; Zhang, H.; Gu, W.; Liu, Y.; Zhang, M. Ginsenoside Rb1 Protects Hippocampal Neurons from High Glucose-induced Neurotoxicity by Inhibiting GSK3β-mediated CHOP Induction. Mol. Med. Rep. 2014, 9, 1434-1438. DOI: 10.3892/mmr.2014.1958

[33] Fujimoto J, Sakaguchi H, Aoki I, Toyoki H, Khatun S & Tamaya T. Inhibitory effect of ginsenoside-Rb2 on invasiveness of uterine endometrial cancer cells to the basement membrane. Eur J. Gynaecol. Oncol. 2001;22:339-341.

[34] Wu J, Yang H, Zhao Q, Zhang X, Lou Y. Ginsenoside Rg1 exerts a protective effect against Aβ25-35-induced toxicity in primary cultured rat cortical neurons through the NF-κB/NO pathway. Int J Mol Med. 2016;37(3):781-788. DOI: 10.3892/ijmm.2016.2485.

[35] Chen WF, Lau WS, Cheung PY, Guo DA, Wong MS. Activation of insulin-like growth factor I

receptor-mediated pathway by ginsenoside Rg1. Br J Pharmacol. 2006 Mar;147(5):542-551. DOI: 10.1038/sj.bjp.0706640.

[36] Zhang X, Shi M, Bjørås M, Wang W, Zhang G, Han J, Liu Z, Zhang Y, Wang B, Chen J, Zhu Y, Xiong L, Zhao G. Ginsenoside Rd promotes glutamate clearance by up-regulating glial glutamate transporter GLT-1 via PI3K/AKT and ERK1/2 pathways. Front Pharmacol. 2013;4:152. DOI: 10.3389/fphar.2013.00152.

[37] Hu G, Wu Z, Yang F, Zhao H, Liu X, Deng Y, Shi M, Zhao G. Ginsenoside Rd blocks AIF mitochondrio-nuclear translocation and NF-κB nuclear accumulation by inhibiting poly(ADP-ribose) polymerase-1 after focal cerebral ischemia in rats. Neurol Sci. 2013;34(12):2101-2106. DOI: 10.1007/s10072-013-1344-6.

[38] Chen L.M., Zhou X.M., Cao Y.L., and Hu W.X. Neuroprotection of ginsenoside Re in cerebral ischemia-reperfusion injury in rats. Journal of Asian Natural Products Research. 2008:10(5), 439-445. DOI: 10.1080/10286020801892292

[39] Kim SW, Kwon HY, Chi DW, Shim JH, Park JD, Lee YH, Pyo S., Rhee DK. Reversal of P- glycoprotein-mediated multidrug resistance by ginsenoside Rg3. Biochem. Pharmacol. 2003;65(1): 75-82. DOI: 10.1016/s0006-2952(02)01446-6

[40] Kim HS, Lee EH, Ko SR, Choi KJ, Park JH., Im DS. Effects of ginsenosides Rg3 and Rh2 on the proliferation of prostate cancer cells. Arch. Pharm. Res. 2004; 27:429-435. DOI: 10.1007/BF02980085

[41] Luo X, Wang CZ, Chen J, Song WX, Luo J, Tang N, He BC, Kang Q, Wang Y, Du W, et al. Characterization of gene expression regulated by American

ginseng and ginsenoside Rg3 in human colorectal cancer cells. Int J Oncol 2008; 32:975-983. DOI: 10.3892/ijo.32.5.975

[42] Surh YJ, Na HK, Lee JY, Keum YS. Molecular mechanisms underlying anti-tumor promoting activities of heat-processed *Panax ginseng* C.A. Meyer. J Korean Med Sci 2001;16:38-41. DOI: 10.3346/jkms.2001.16.S.S38

[43] Zheng G., Wang J. Protein Regulating Networks underlying Multiple Actions against Cancer Delivered by Ginseng. 2018 IEEE International Conference on Bioinformatics and Biomedicine (BIBM). 2018;1977-1981.

[44] Yan J, Ma Y., Zhao F., Gu W., Jiao Y. Identification of Immunomodulatory Signatures Induced by American Ginseng in Murine Immune Cells. Evidence-Based Complementary and Alternative Medicine. Volume 2013, Article ID 972814, 1-12. DOI:10.1155/2013/972814

[45] Joob B, Wiwanitkit V. Combination between ginseng and arginine regimen: Is there any synergistic effect? J Med Trop 2016;18:18-21. DOI: 10.4103/2276-7096.176048

[46] Ong Lai Teik D, Lee XS, Lim CJ, Low CM, Muslima M, Aquili L. Ginseng and *Ginkgo biloba* Effects on Cognition as Modulated by Cardiovascular Reactivity: A Randomised Trial. PLoS One. 2016;11(3):e0150447. DOI: 10.1371/journal.pone.0150447.

[47] Diana A, Michielin O, Zoete V. SwissTargetPrediction: updated data and new features for efficient prediction of protein targets of small molecules. Nucleic Acids Research. 2019;1-8. DOI: 10.1093/nar/gkz382

[48] Clarke, D.J.B.; Kuleshov, M.V.; Schilder, B.M.; Torre, D.; Duffy, M.E.; Keenan, A.B.; Lachmann, A.; Feldmann A.S.; Gundersen G.W.;

Silverstein M.C.; Wang Z.; Ma'ayan A. eXpression2Kinases (X2K) Web: linking expression signatures to upstream cell signaling networks. Nucleic Acids Res. 2018, 46, W1: 171-179. DOI:10.1093/nar/gky458

[49] Zhang H, Abid S, Ahn J.C, Mathiyalagan R, Kim Y-J, Yang D-C, and Wang Y, (2020). Characteristics of *Panax ginseng* Cultivars in Korea and China. Molecules 2020, 25, 2635; DOI:10.3390/molecules25112635

[50] Wang N., Wang X., He M., Zheng W., et al. Network pharmacology-based active compounds and pharmacological mechanisms of ginseng for depression in post-COVID-19. Research Square, 2020;1-12. DOI:10.21203/rs.3.rs-40858/v1

[51] Bin Sayeed MS, Karim SMR, Sharmin T, and Morshed MM. Critical Analysis on Characterization, Systemic Effect, and Therapeutic Potential of Beta-Sitosterol: A Plant-Derived Orphan Phytosterol. Medicines 2016, 3, 29; DOI: 10.3390/medicines3040029

Chapter 6

Ginseng in Hair Growth and Viability

Mercedes De Mirecki-Garrido, Ruymán Santana-Farré,
Noelia Guedes-Hernandez, Francisco Jimenez-Acosta
and Dionisio L. Lorenzo-Villegas

Abstract

The hair follicle is the unique organ that has the capacity of undergoing cyclic transformations following periods of growth (anagen), regression (catagen), and rest (telogen) regenerating itself to restart the cycle. The dynamic capacity of hair to growth and rest enables mammals to control hair growth and length in different body side and to change their coats. Unlike what is observed in many animals in which the pelage synchronously passes from one phase of the cycle to other all stages of growth cycle are simultaneously found in the human pelage, the growth pattern is a mosaic where the hair cycling staging of one hair root is completely independent of it nearest hair follicle, meaning that each follicular unit (FU) can contain follicles in different stages at any given time. A variety of factors, such as nutritional status, hormones, exposure to radiations, chemotherapy or radiotherapy, environmental pollution or drugs may affect hair growth, and affects the number of hairs, this progressive hair loss has a cosmetic and social impact that often significantly affects social and psychological well-being of the patient that suffers from this hair loss. Although a number of therapies, such as finasteride and minoxidil, are approved medications, a wide variety of classes of phytochemicals and natural products, including those present in ginseng are being testing. The purpose of this chapter is to focus on study the potential of ginseng and its metabolites in hair loss.

Keywords: Ginseng, Hair, Hair Follicle, Hair growth, Hair Viability

1. Introduction

1.1 Hair structure

Hair is made of several proteins, the principal protein that compound the fibrous structure of the hair is keratin, in addition to keratin, which has a high content of the amino acid cysteine, the hair also contains water, lipids, minerals, and the pigment melanin.

The hair shaft (the visible fiber that is growth above the skin), is a fiber with a variety of color depending of the melanin content that pigmented the keratin fiber. The dermal element in the hair follicle is the dermal papilla, which is majorly former by fibroblast cells, this dermal element controls the hair cycle.

The fiber of the hair, the hair shaft, grows from the hair follicle which is a tubular structure that forms a bulb around the matrix of the hair bulb, specialized dermal stem cell and different types of keratinocytes, from this hair bulb that form the dermal papilla the hair shaft growth by division of proliferative cells, thus cells goes to a process of differentiated, keratinized, and pigmented in the hair follicle to form the hair shaft in a cycling manner. The diameter of the hair shaft is directly related to the size of the papilla, and allows us to define the miniaturized hairs and normal hair.

The hair structure is composed by concentric layers that forms the hair follicle, the medulla which is the center is includes the cortex and outwards the cuticle of the cortex, and is surrounded by the inner and outer root sheath, and all the mini-organ is surrounded by connective tissue.

1.2 Hair function

The functional aspect of hair is not only to protect from radiation, heat or cold and any extern agent but also contribute to the appearance and personality. The loss of the hair contributes to psychological, social and psychosocial problems, generating a cosmetic and social impact in our society.

1.3 Hair cycle

The hair follicle has the unique capacity of undergoing periods of growth (anagen), regression (catagen), and rest (telogen and exogen) before regenerating itself to restart the cycle [1–4] (**Figure 1**). This dynamic cycling capacity enables mammals to change their coats, and for hair length to be controlled on different body sites [5].

Unlike what is observed in many animals in which the pelage synchronously passes from one phase of the cycle to other all stages of growth cycle are simultaneously found in the human, the growth pattern is a mosaic where the hair cycling staging of one hair root is completely independent of it nearest hair follicle, meaning that each follicular unit (FU) can contain follicles in different stages at any given time. In healthy individuals, 80–90% of follicles are in the anagen phase, 1–2% in the catagen phase, and 10–15% in the telogen phase [6]. The hair grows around one centimeter a month, and has a variable growth speed being faster in the summer than in winter. The growth phase, or anagen phase, lasts an average of 3–5 years. This normal hair-growth cycle can be modified or by internal or external factors such as hormones, stress, sun, disease, exposure to environmental pollution, drugs and smoking. This changes in the growth cycle and quality of hair can leads to hair loss by a shortening of the anagen phase, a premature ingression of the catagen phase, the prolongation of the telogen phase or a loss of the hair

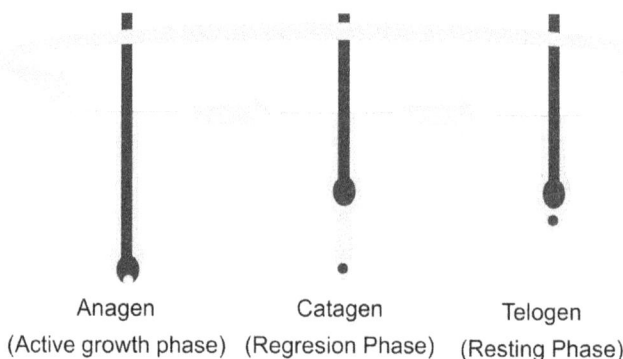

Anagen Catagen Telogen
(Active growth phase) (Regresion Phase) (Resting Phase)

Figure 1.
Hair cycle stages scheme, phase of growth (anagen), regression (catagen), and rest (telogen) before regenerating itself to restart the cycle.

follicle function [6, 7]. Common hair loss is medically named as alopecia, and can be suffer by men and women.

1.4 Hair loss

Research has shown that in hair loss, the percentage of telogen follicles is increased, while the percentage of anagen and catagen follicles is reduced. A healthy individual loses approximately 100–150 hairs per day [6]. Cell-signaling pathways in hair follicular cells resulting in the induction of apoptosis, changes in usual pattern of hair cycling, inducing the hair follicle to turn into regression or resting phase and thinning or fracture of the hair shaft leads to progressive hair loss and alopecia [7].

Hair loss is a universal problem for numerous people in the world, is a disorder in which the hair falls out from skin areas such as scalp, the body and face. Multiples factors contribute to hair loss including genetics, hormones, nutritional status, and environmental exposure (exposure to radiations, environmental toxicants...), medications and nutrition.

Androgenic alopecia can be suffered by women and men and the androgens hormones are the most important of the factors that cause the hair lost patron characterized by a miniaturized of the hair follicles that leads to hair lost in the frontal to parietal area.

Other forms of hair loss are for example caused by immunogenic hair loss, like alopecia areata, this is characterized by a spot of hair lost all around the scalp. The approved therapies such as finasteride and minoxidil, are the traditional medication used for this hair lost diseases, a few others are in progress, like a wide variety of diverse phytochemicals, including those present in ginseng, the ginsenosides which have demonstrated hair growth-promoting effects in a large number of preclinical studies [7].

Androgenic baldness (androgenic alopecia) and circular/spot baldness (alopecia areata) are the most common forms of hair loss. The first is characterized by high sensitivity of the hair follicles to DH, while the second is induced by an autoimmune reaction [8, 9]. Hair also possesses its own immune system, the failure of which can lead to spot baldness (alopecia areata).

Alopecia is extended all round the world, reaching nowadays approximately to 10 million patients suffering from alopecia. Considering the pathological background of alopecia and its impact on an individual's health and social value, there is now a growing interest in the development of novel therapeutics for its medical management [7].

1.5 Conventional treatment for hair lost

Given the negative psychosocial impact of hair loss, patients follow different therapies, conventional treatments such as the two medications approved by the United States Food and Drug Administration (US-FDA): Minoxidil and Finasteride, for the treatment of alopecia.

Finasteride has a potent effect against androgens, being non-steroidal, it has shown to prevent male and female hair loss through the inhibition of type II 5α-reductase, which affects androgen metabolism avoiding the conversion of free testosterone into 5α-dihydrotestosterone, playing an important role in the pathogenesis of androgenetic alopecia in men and women [10].

The effect of minoxidil as hair growth stimulating has been known over last decades, since it was introduced in the early 1970 as a treatment for hypertension. But yet the basic mechanism of action on the hair follicle is not clearly understood [11, 12].

These drugs work improving the quality of the hair follicles and reducing the hair lost but exhibit certain adverse effects, such as allergic contact dermatitis, erythema, and itching, and also stop recommended guideline of minoxidil leads to recurrence of alopecia and a prolonged use of finasteride causes male sexual dysfunction and appears as a major cause of infertility and teratogenicity in females.

Patient that do not see significant hair restoration with conventional therapies or suffer side effects often change from these conventional treatments to alternative medicine trying new treatments from the vast resources of natural products, in an attempt to find safe, natural and efficacious therapies to restore the hair.

2. Natural products

Natural products as it is known in the market "Dietary supplements" includes diverse subgroups like vitamins, probiotics, minerals, herbs, extracts, gels that do not require Food and Drug Administration (FDA) approval [13].

To treat hair loss are available treatments using amino acids, caffeine, capsaicin, curcumin, garlic gel, onion gel and extract, cinnamon, *Aloe Vera* gel, marine proteins, melatonin, procyanidin, pumpkin seed oil, rosemary oil, saw palmetto, vitamin B7 (biotin), vitamin D, vitamin E, zinc and Ginseng [9, 13].

3. Ginseng

Ginseng is an ancient herbal remedy that was recorded in The Herbal Classic of the Divine Plowman, the oldest comprehensive Materia Medica, which was scripted approximately 2000 years ago [9].

Among different species which are known as ginseng, *Panax ginseng* (Korean or Asian red ginseng) is the most frequently used one. The Ginseng is widely appreciated because it promotes health effect improving the immune response, the cardiovascular system, helping with sexual dysfunctions, preventing cancer, inhibiting tumor cell proliferation among others. In Dermatologic diseases, cancer is being investigate for its therapeutic effects in skin wound reparation, reducing immune response in dermatitis, reduces and prevent skin damage due to photo aging and cold hypersensitivity, improves hair growth reducing hair loss in alopecia [14].

Nowadays has gained fame as one of the most popular herbs originating from Eastern Countries, because contemporary science has revealed that ginseng contains a wide variety of bioactive constituents, especially a group of saponin compounds collectively known as ginsenosides, which have been proposed to account for most of the diverse biological activities, including the hair-growth potential of ginseng [9]. Ginsenosides can be classified, depending on the number of hydroxyl groups available for glycosylation via dehydration reactions, as protopanaxadiol (PPD) and protopanaxatriol (PPT). Common PPD-type ginsenosides include ginsenosides Rb1, Rb2, Rc, Rd., Rg3, F2, Rh2, compound K (cK), and PPD, whereas PPT-type ginsenosides include Re, Rf, Rg1, Rg2, F1, Rh1, and PPT [9] and malony ginsenosides mRb1, mRb2 and mRbc [15]. Ginseng extract or its specific ginsenosides have been tested for their potential to promote hair growth.

3.1 Ginseng biochemical effects on hair growth promotion

The major bioactive constituents of ginseng are ginsenosides and there has been evidences suggesting that promote hair growth by enhancing proliferation of dermal papilla and preventing hair loss via modulation of various cell-signaling pathways [9, 16, 17].

The role of 5α-reductase enzyme in the hair-loss process has been well-documented [18], affects androgen metabolism, and it is the pathway how drugs approved are used nowadays.

Novel therapeutics ways for the management of hair loss and alopecia improving hair-follicle proliferation and reducing hair-loss need new targets (**Figure 2**). These targets include, matrix metalloproteinases (MMPs), extracellular signal-regulated protein kinase (ERK), and Janus-activated kinase (JAK), the activation of the pro-liferation by WNT/Dickkopf homolog 1 (DKK1), sonic hedgehog (Shh), vascular endothelial growth factor (VEGF), apoptosis inhibition by transforming growth factor-beta (TGF-β).

3.1.1 Photo aging prevention

Photo aging is skin damage induced by radiation exposure (Sun exposure) characterized by different inflammatory responses to ultraviolet radiation (UVR). Excessive UV irradiation is known to cause skin photo damage by release of oxidative species which leads to skin inflammation, and keratinocyte cell death producing photo aging and carcinogenesis.

There are evidences that suggest that misbalances in the hair-growth cycle, affecting keratinocyte and dermal papilla growth [19] is cause by UVR exposure not only producing the damage of the hair shaft as an extracellular tissue, as it is clearly evident but also alters the molecular growth [19].

The Reactive Oxidative Species (ROS) accumulation and activation of matrix metalloproteinase (MMPs), a tissue-degrading enzymes, produced by UV irradiation compromises dermal and epidermal structural integrity [9].

The inhibitory effect of ginsenosides on UVB-induced activation of MMP2 suggests the potential of these ginseng saponins in hair-growth regulation [9]. Ginsenosides Rb2 [20] and 20 (S) PPD, have been reported to reduce the formation of ROS and MMP-2 secretion in cultured human keratinocytes (HaCaT) cells after exposure to UVB radiation. Ginsenoside Rg3 20 (S), reduced ROS generation in

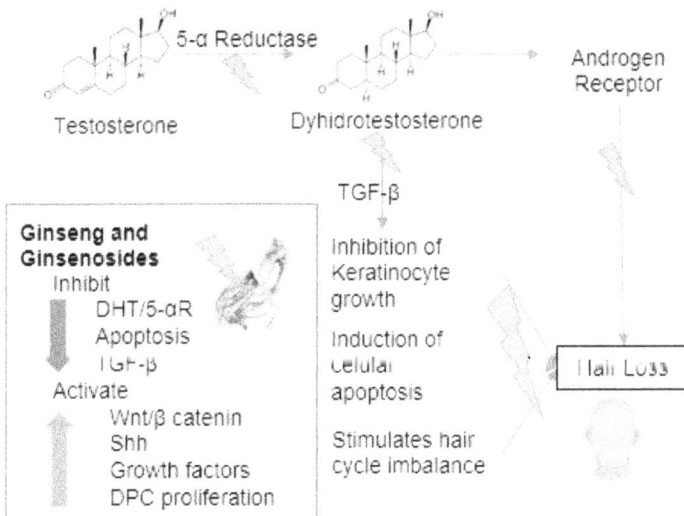

Figure 2.
The effect of the 5α-reductase enzyme, dihydrotestosterone, and the growth factor TGF-β on hair loss and the potential targets of ginseng in hair growth and loss.

HaCaT cells and human dermal fibroblasts without affecting cell viability. The 20 (S) Rg3 also attenuated UVB-induced MMP-2 levels in HaCaT cells [21]. Ginsenoside Rh2 reduced UVB radiation-induced expression and activity of MMP-2 in HaCaT cells, but UVB-induced ROS formation was only suppressed by 20 (S)-Rh2 [22].

Ginsenosides extracts from the Ginseng radix have shown attenuates radiation-induced cell death in the skin, improving hair growth. Ki67 positive number of cells and Bcl2 protein expression, an antiapoptotic protein, are induced by Total-root saponins and ginsenoside Rb1 diminishing apoptotic cells in UVB-exposed human keratinocytes [9, 23]. Ginsenoside F1, an enzymatically modified derivative of ginsenoside Rg1, by maintaining a constant level of the antiapoptotic protein Bcl-2 expression in UVB-irradiated HaCaT cells, protect keratinocytes from radiation-induced apoptosis [9, 24].

3.1.2 Ginsenosides reduces skin aging

Skin aging is a multifactorial process consisting of two distinct and independent mechanisms: intrinsic and extrinsic aging.

Ginsenosides, extracted from Ginseng have been tested in several studies in antiaging [25, 26]. This antiaging effects, of ginseng extract and ginsenosides is produced by maintaining skin structural integrity and regulating hair-growth by stimulating wound healing cells, collagen and hyaluronic acid.

Lee et all incubates fibroblasts, which are key wound-healing cells, with *Panax ginseng*, and found that *P. ginseng* stimulated human dermal fibroblast proliferation and collagen synthesis [27]. Human dermal fibroblast have different functions and are classified as key wound-healing cells because their function includes the production of collagen, growth factors, antioxidants and a balance of matrix-producing proteins and protease enzymes. In the Human fibroblast *P. ginseng* root extract activates human collagen A2 promotes and induces type-1 pro-collagen via phosphorylation of Smad2 [28].

Wrinkle formation, is associated as marker of dermal aging and present a reduced level of hyaluronan in the dermis [29]. On HaCaT cell treated with major ginseng metabolite (compound K, 20-O-beta-D-glucopyranosyl-20 (S)-protopanaxadiol) were report that hyaluronan synthase2 (HAS2) gene is one of the most significantly induced genes [30] and also was tested that topical application of compound K on mouse skin and shows elevated the expression of hyaluronan synthase-2 [30]. The hyaluronan synthase-2 is an enzyme essential to hyaluronan synthesis, hyaluronan is a major component of most extracellular matrices that has a structural role in tissues architectures and regulates cell adhesion, migration and differentiation.

These antiaging effects of ginseng extracts through Src kinase-dependent activation of ERK and AKT/PKB kinases in the dermis and papillary dermis result in improved skin health, thereby ensuring hair-follicle health and a regular hair cycle [9, 30].

3.1.3 Ginseng on androgen alopecia

The exposure to androgens is the major triggers for hair loss is which in most cases is genetically predetermined in androgenic alopecia patients [9, 31, 32].

The androgen that mainly plays a role in altering hair cycling is 5α-dihydrotestosterone (DHT), which is a metabolite of testosterone. The conversion of testosterone to DHT is mediated by the 5α-reductase (5αR) enzyme in each follicle [33, 34] (**Figure 2**). Treatment with 5α-reductase inhibitors, e.g., finasteride, prevents the development of alopecia and increases scalp-hair growth [9].

Topical application of ginseng extract or ginsenosides was reported to enhance hair growth. Rhizomes of *P. ginseng* (red ginseng) containing a considerable amount of ginsenoside Ro, Ro is the predominant ginsenoside in the rhizome showed greater dose-dependent inhibitory effects against testosterone 5α-reductase (5αR) [35]. Ginsenoside Rg3 (a unique ginsenoside in red ginseng) and Rd. also exhibited similar inhibitory effects against 5αR [36]. Another variety of ginseng, the Parribacus japonicas rhizome extract that contains a larger quantity of ginsenoside Ro also inhibited 5αR enzyme activity. Topical administration of red-ginseng rhizome extracts and ginsenoside Ro onto shaved skin of C57BL/6 mice abrogated testosterone-mediated suppression of hair regrowth [36].

Major components of hair regenerative capacity such as linoleic acid (LA) and β-sitosterol (SITOS) were significantly restored with Red Ginseng Oil (RGO) after testosterone (TES)-induced delay of anagen entry in C57BL/6 mice, also RGO and its major components reduced the protein level of TGF-β and enhanced the expression of anti-apoptotic protein Bcl-2, suggesting that RGO is a potent novel therapeutic natural product for treatment of androgenic alopecia [37].

Red Ginseng Extract (RGE) and ginsenosides protect hair matrix keratinocyte proliferation against dihydrotestosterone (DHT)-induced suppression and affects the expression of androgen receptor.

Moreover, RGE, ginsenoside-Rb1, and ginsenoside-Rg3 at lower levels that have been shown to inhibit 5a-reductase [35] inhibit the DHT-induced suppression of hair matrix keratinocyte proliferation and the DHT-induced upregulation of the mRNA expression of androgen receptor in hDPCs [16]. DHT is the product of testosterone and does not require the activity of 5a-reductase to affect hair follicles, and the inhibitory effect of DHT on hair growth is mediated by the androgen receptor in DPCs [38]. These results suggest that red ginseng may promote hair growth in humans through the regulation of androgen receptor signaling [16].

3.1.4 Effects of ginsenosides on chemotherapy

Majeed et al. review the recent perspectives of ginseng phytochemicals as therapeutics in oncology and explain the chemotherapeutic effect of ginsenoside as result of its appetites, ant proliferative, anti-angiogenic, anti-inflammatory and anti-oxidant properties [39]. The anticancer effect of ginseng was proven in various types of cancer: breast, lung, liver, colon and skin cancer. It increases the mitochondrial accumulation of apoptosis protein and down regulate the expression of anti-apoptotic protein, reducing cancer development. It also aids in the reduction of alopecia, fatigue and nausea, the known side effects of chemotherapeutic drugs [39].

Alopecia induced by chemotherapy is one of the most distressing side effects for patients undergoing chemotherapy. One drug used as chemotherapy is Cyclophosphamide (CP), also known as cytophosphane. Cyclophosphamide metabolite, 4-hydroperoxycyclophosphamide (4-HC) inhibited human hair growth, induced premature catagen development, and inhibited proliferation and stimulated apoptosis of hair matrix keratinocytes inducing the side effect of alopecia. In human hair follicle organ culture model pre-treatment with Korean Red Ginseng (KRG) before cyclophosphamide metabolite Dong In Keum et all shows that KRG suppress 4-HC-induced inhibition of matrix keratinocyte proliferation and stimulation of matrix keratinocyte apoptosis, playing a protective effect on 4-HC-induced hair growth inhibition and premature catagen development. Moreover, KRG restored 4-HC-induced p53 and Bax/Bcl2 expression [17].

3.1.5 Activation of dermal papillary cell proliferation

Different intracellular signaling pathways are involving and plays a critical role in stimulating hair growth by promoting dermal papillary-cell proliferation.

Hair growth is promote by Ginsenoside Rg3 upregulating Vascular Endothelial Growth Factor (VEGF) expression [36]. VEGF is a signaling protein which is released from the epithelium and increases the angiogenesis of the hair follicle [9, 40–42]. Was also demonstrate by Shin et al. that Rg3 increased the proliferation of human dermal papillary cells, associating this proliferation with an upregulation of mRNA expression of VEGF also stimulated stem cells by upregulating factor-activating CD34 and CD8 [36] and promoted hair growth even more than minoxidil in mouse [43] it was conclude that Rg3 might increase hair growth through stimulation of hair follicle stem cells [36].

RGE and ginsenoside-Rb1 enhanced the proliferation of hair matrix keratino-cytes, human hair-follicle dermal papillary cells (hDPCs). Treated hair with RGE or ginsenoside-Rb1 exhibited substantial cell proliferation and the associated phos-phorylation of ERK and AKT [16], it was recently demonstrated that ERK activation plays an important role in the proliferation of hDPCs [42] and AKT mediates critical signals for cell survival and also regulates the survival of DPCs as an antiapoptotic molecule [9, 16, 44] proliferation and the prolongation of the survival in the hDPCs by red ginseng may be mediated by the ERK and AKT signaling pathway [9, 16].

Human DPC treatment with Gintonin-enriched fraction (GEF) stimulated vascular endothelial growth factor release. Topical application of GEF and minoxidil promoted hair growth in a dose-dependent manner. Histological analysis showed that GEF and minoxidil increased the number of hair follicles and hair weight [45].

The Bcl-2 family proteins is notable for their regulation of apoptosis machinery, a form of programmed cell death, the member of this family either acts as antiapop-totic or pro apoptotic in nature. During the hair cycle, the dermal papillary cells (DPC) is the only region where Bcl-2 is expressed consistently and is considered to resist apoptosis [9, 46–48]. In mice Fructus *Panax ginseng* extract (FPG) increases the expression of Bcl-2 and decreases Bax expression, a pro apoptotic species, in cultured DPCs [49]. Parks et all concluded that FPG extract improves the cell prolif-eration of human DPCs through anti apoptotic activation. Topical administration of FPG extract might have hair regeneration activity for the treatment of hair loss [49].

3.1.6 Modulation of Wnt/Dickkopf homolog 1 (DKK1), sonic hedgehog (Shh), JAK-STAT3 and TGF-β signaling by ginseng

Shh/Gli and Wnt/β path way and related proteins (Shh (Sonic hedgehog,) Smoothened (Smo), β-catenin, Cyclin D1 Cyclin E and Gli1 (glioma-associated oncogene homolog)) are associated to hair regeneration, promoting telogen-to-anagen transition, hair follicle formation and growth [50–56].

Wingless-type integration-site (WNT) signaling plays a key role in hair-follicle development. Activation of WNT signaling is necessary for initiation of follicular develop, the blockade of WNT signaling by overexpression of the WNT inhibitor, Dickkopf Homolog 1 (DKK1), prevents hair-follicle formation in mice [50] and inhibited hair growth [9, 50].

β-catenin signaling is essential for epithelial stem-cell fate since keratinocytes adopt an epidermal fate in the absence of β-catenin [51], and this signaling pathway is related to WNT [52] affecting hair follicle placodes formation, when β-catenin is mutated dur-ing embryogenesis, formation of placodes that generate hair follicles is blocked [53].

The role of TGF-β in hair loss has been documented through the study revealing that treatment with a TGF-β antagonist can promote hair growth via preventing catagen progression [57]. Also through the activation of TGF-β and brain-derived neurotrophic factor (BDNF), it was describe that it was enhanced the transition from the anagen to the catagen phase [58].

Since TGF-β1 induces catagen in hair follicles and it is closely related to alopecia progression it can be say that acts as a pathogenic mediator of androgenic alopecia [57, 59] and red ginseng extract can delay the catagen phase and holds the potential to promote hair growth, thought downregulation or inhibition of the TGF-β pathway.

On Young Go Kim investigation was concluded that on ultraviolet B (UVB)-irradiated skin aging in mice, oral administration of Red Ginseng extract protects from skin damage induced by ultraviolet B (UVB)-irradiation, increases of skin thickness and pigmentation, reduction of skin elasticity, inhibited the increases of epidermis and corium thickness. The administration of Red Ginseng extract exert the protective action on UVB-radiation skin aging inhibiting the increase of skin TGF-beta1 content induced by UVB irradiation [60].

Furthermore on Zheng Li the hair-growth-promoting effects of Protopanaxatiol type ginsenoside Re were associated with the downregulation of TGF-β-pathway-related genes, which are involved in the control of hair-growth phase-transition-related signaling pathways [61]. On their study shows that topical administration of ginsenoside Re on to the back skin of nude mice for up to 45 days significantly increased hair-shaft length and hair existent time, and stimulated hair-shaft elongation in the ex vivo cultures of hair follicles isolated from C57BL/6 mouse [61].

The hyper activation of the c-Jun-N-terminal kinase (JNK) pathway in associate with an activation of TGF-β-induced hair loss. Korean red ginseng has been attributed to exert protective effects onTGF-β-induced hair loss by the inhibition of JNK on radiation-induced apoptosis of HaCaT cells [62].

By promoting telogen-to-anagen transition of follicular cells and epidermal growth, Shh/Gli regulates hair-follicle development, growth and cycling [54, 55]. Shh$^{-/-}$ mice develop have abnormal hair follicular cells in the dermal papillae and blocking Shh activity mice diminished hair growth, this results indicates the importance of Shh signaling in hair-growth promotion [56].

Androgenetic alopecia is related to testosterone (TES)-induced delay of anagen phase and hair loss. In C57BL/6 mice Red-ginseng oil (RGO) reversed testosterone-induced suppression of hair regeneration through early inducing anagen phase by up-regulating the expression of Shh/Gliand Wnt/β pathway-related proteins, Shh, Smoothened (Smo), β-catenin, Cyclin D1 Cyclin E and Gli1. Additionally, RGO reduced the protein level of TGF-β but enhanced the expression of anti-apoptotic protein Bcl-2 [37] suggesting that RGO is a potent therapeutic natural product for treatment of androgenic alopecia possibly through hair re-growth activity [37].

The signaling pathway and anagen induction effect of ginsenoside F2 were investigated and compared with finasteride on the effect of hair growth induction in Heon-Sub Shin at all paper [43] where MTT assay results indicated cell proliferation in human DPC increased a 30% with ginsenoside F2 treatment compared to finasteride [43]. Studding the expression of β-catenin and its transcriptional coactivator Lef-1, the Ginsenoside F2 compared to finasteride group, increased the expressions while decreased the expression of DKK-1. Tissue histological analysis shows that administration of ginsenoside F2 promoted hair growth as compared to finasteride, increase in the number of hair follicles, thickness of the epidermis, and follicles of the anagen phase [43]. Heon-Sub Shin conclude that ginsenoside F2 might be a potential new therapeutic compound for anagen induction and hair growth through the Wnt signal pathway [43]. In another study by Matsuda et al., ginsenosides Rg3 and Rb1 [63] extracted from red ginseng stimulates hair growth activity in an organ culture of mouse vibrissa follicles. No detailed explanations are given in this paper about the mechanism of hair growth, but the results presented by Matsuda et al. [63] indicated that Ginseng Radix possesses hair growth promoting activity.

Panax ginseng (PG) has diverse pharmacological effects such as anti-aging and anti-inflammation it exert this effects thought stimulating the proliferation and inhibiting the apoptosis [64]. PG extract treatment affected the expression of apoptosis-related genes in HFs, Bcl-2 and Bax, through this regulation reversed the effect of DKK-1 on ex vivo human hair organ culture, antagonizes DKK-1-induced catagen-like changes [9, 64].

Growth factors and cytokines have been proved to influence hair follicle development or cycling [65] overexpression and/or secretion of Cytokines, such as interleukins (ILs) and interferons (IFN), cause skin inflammation, TGF beta 1 partially inhibited hair growth and EGF, TNF alpha and IL-1 beta completely abrogated it [66]. There is an aberrant expression pattern of cytokines in alopecia areata hair follicles.

The presence of CD8+ T cells and NKG2D+ cells around the peri-bulbar area of the affected hair follicles [67] and upregulation of several ILs, such as IL-2, IL-7, IL-15, and IL-21, and IFN-γ leads to immune activation area where're main suppressed natural killer (NK) cells [68] and is defined as immune-tolerated area. Loss of immune tolerance [68] or immune activation [67], leads to hair-follicle dystrophy and acceleration of the catagen phase [9] by the activation of a cytotoxic cluster of differentiation 8-positive (CD8+) and NK group 2D-positive (NKG2D+) T cells. In alopecia Areata (AA) are found more CD57 – CD16+ NK cells and there is a association between NK cells and the collapse of HF-IP (immune privilege) while normal human scalp skin— that indeed there is no sign of an NK attack on normal anagen VI HFs [69].

Phosphorylate Stat3 in the Janus Kinase (JAK)/Signal transducer and activator of transcription-3 (STAT3) pathway regulate the activation of CD8+ and the NKG2D+ CD8+ T cells [70]. The inhibition of the upstream pathway JAK appears as a plausible target for developing a therapy for hair loss [67]. In fact, a number of JAK inhibitors, such as tofacitinib, ruxolitinib, baricitinib, CTP-543, PF-06651600 and PF-06700841 are in the progress of developing a therapy for alopecia [71, 72] more often in alopecia areata a common form of non-scarring hair loss that usually starts abruptly with a very high psychological impact [73], it is a T-cell-mediated disease which produces circular patches of non-scarring hair loss and nail dystrophy [72].

Ginsenoside Rk1 inhibited the lipopolysaccharide- stimulated phosphorylation of JAK2 and STAT3 in murine macrophage cells [74] and Ginsenoside 20(S)-Rh2 exerts anti-cancer activity through targeting IL-6-induced JAK2/STAT3 [75]. Topical application of ginsenoside F2 by inhibiting the production of IL-17 and ROS, ameliorated dermal inflammation skin [69]. In the pathogenesis of alopecia areata is believed to be an imbalance of inflammatory cytokines IL-17. Monoclonal antibodies against IL-17A leads to hair regrowth in human volunteers [76]. Treatment with *Panax ginseng* saponins diminished the proliferation and differentiation of Th17 cells and decreased IL-17 expression [77]. This regulating IL-17 secretion ginsenosides may enhance hair growth in alopecia areata [69, 77]. It would be interesting to investigate whether ginsenoside Rk1 or other ginsenosides can target JAK/STAT3 signaling in dermal papilla and diminish activation of inflammation and immune cells.

4. Conclusion

Ginseng may be a multipurpose natural medicine with an extended history of medical application throughout the globe, particularly in Eastern countries.

The beneficial effects of Ginseng cover a good spectrum from immune to cardiovascular, cancer and sexual diseases. New advances in the science leads elucidate new pharmacological activity of the ginseng and its ginsenosides. There are some studies of the use of Ginseng in dermatology investigating its effects from molecular to physiological in a skin cancer, dermatitis, alopecia wound injury and of course hair loss because also ginseng and its ginsenosides regulate the expression and activity of major proteins involved in hair-cycling phases, so the medical use of ginseng is not only restricted to the improvement of general wellness, but also extended to the treatment of organ-specific pathological conditions, like hair.

Ginseng and its metabolites are associate with the induction of anagen phase preventing hair lost and promoting hair growth although further studies should be done to elucidate and clarified the mechanisms by which ginseng and its metabolites regulate human hair health.

Conflict of interest

The authors declare no conflict of interest.

Acronyms and abbreviations

AA	Alopecia Areata
AGA	Androgenetic Alopecia
FU	Follicular Unit
US-FDA	United States Food and Drug Administration
DKK1	Dickkopf homolog 1
Shh	sonic hedgehog
VEGF	vascular endothelial growth factor
TGF-β	transforming growth factor-beta
MMPs	matrix metalloproteinase
ERK	extracellular signal-regulated protein kinase
JAK	Janus-activated kinase
PPD	protopanaxadiol
PPT	protopanaxatriol
cK	compound K
UVR	ultraviolet radiation
ROS	reactive oxygen species
LA	linoleic acid
SITOS	β-sitosterol
TES	testosterone
HHDPCs	human hair-follicle dermal papillary cells
RGE	rcd-ginseng extract
HFDPCs	hair follicle dermal papilla cells
GEF	Gintonin-enriched fraction
KRG	Korean Red Ginseng
DPCs	Dermal papillary cells
NKG2D+	NK group 2D-positive
ULBP3	UL16-binding protein 3
Shh/Gli	glioma-associated oncogene homolog
CD8+	cluster of differentiation 8-positive
ILs	interleukins
IFN	interferons
ORS	outer root sheath
STAT3	Signal transducer and activator of transcription-3
WNT	Wingless-type integration-site
GEF	Gintonin-enriched fraction

Author details

Mercedes De Mirecki-Garrido[1,2*], Ruymán Santana-Farré[1],
Noelia Guedes-Hernandez[2], Francisco Jimenez-Acosta[1,2]
and Dionisio L. Lorenzo-Villegas[1]

1 Faculty of Health Sciences, University Fernando Pessoa Canarias,
Las Palmas de Gran Canaria, Spain

2 Mediteknia Skin and Hair Laboratory, Las Palmas de Gran Canaria, Spain

*Address all correspondence to: mdemirecki@ufpcanarias.es

IntechOpen

References

[1] Chandrashekar BS, Nandhini T, Vasanth V, Sriram R, Navale S. Topical minoxidil fortified with finasteride: An account of maintenance of hair density after replacing oral finasteride. Indian dermatology online journal. 2015;6(1): 17-20.

[2] Rossi A, Anzalone A, Fortuna MC, Caro G, Garelli V, Pranteda G, et al. Multi-therapies in androgenetic alopecia: review and clinical experiences. Dermatologic therapy. 2016;29(6):424-32.

[3] Chase HB. Growth of the hair. Physiol Rev. 1954;34(1):113-26.

[4] Kligman AM. The human hair cycle. J Invest Dermatol. 1959;33:307-16.

[5] Van Scott EJ, Reinertson RP, Steinmuller R. The growing hair roots of the human scalp and morphologic changes therein following amethopterin therapy. J Invest Dermatol. 1957;29(3): 197-204.

[6] Paus R, Cotsarelis G. The biology of hair follicles. N Engl J Med. 1999;341(7): 491-7.

[7] Higgins CA, Westgate GE, Jahoda CA. From telogen to exogen: mechanisms underlying formation and subsequent loss of the hair club fiber. The Journal of investigative dermatology. 2009;129(9):2100-8.

[8] Zgonc Skulj A, Poljsak N, Kocevar Glavac N, Kreft S. Herbal preparations for the treatment of hair loss. Archives of dermatological research. 2020;312(6):395-406.

[9] Choi BY. Hair-Growth Potential of Ginseng and Its Major Metabolites: A Review on Its Molecular Mechanisms. International journal of molecular sciences. 2018;19(9).

[10] Thigpen AE, Davis DL, Milatovich A, Mendonca BB, Imperato-McGinley J, Griffin JE, et al. Molecular genetics of steroid 5 alpha-reductase 2 deficiency. J Clin Invest. 1992;90(3): 799-809.

[11] Messenger AG, Rundegren J. Minoxidil: mechanisms of action on hair growth. Br J Dermatol. 2004;150(2): 186-94.

[12] Hoffmann R, Happle R. Current understanding of androgenetic alopecia. Part I: etiopathogenesis. Eur J Dermatol. 2000;10(4):319-27.

[13] Hosking AM, Juhasz M, Atanaskova Mesinkovska N. Complementary and Alternative Treatments for Alopecia: A Comprehensive Review. Skin appendage disorders. 2019;5(2):72-89.

[14] Sabouri-Rad S, Sabouri-Rad S, Sahebkar A, Tayarani-Najaran Z. Ginseng in Dermatology: A Review. Curr Pharm Des. 2017;23(11):1649-66.

[15] Chuang WC, Wu HK, Sheu SJ, Chiou SH, Chang HC, Chen YP. A comparative study on commercial samples of ginseng radix. Planta Med. 1995;61(5):459-65.

[16] Park GH, Park KY, Cho HI, Lee SM, Han JS, Won CH, et al. Red ginseng extract promotes the hair growth in cultured human hair follicles. J Med Food. 2015;18(3):354-62.

[17] Keum DI, Pi LQ, Hwang ST, Lee WS. Protective effect of Korean Red Ginseng against chemotherapeutic drug-induced premature catagen development assessed with human hair follicle organ culture model. J Ginseng Res. 2016;40(2):169-75.

[18] Inui S, Itami S. Androgen actions on the human hair follicle: perspectives. Exp Dermatol. 2013;22(3):168-71.

[19] Rattan SI, Kryzch V, Schnebert S, Perrier E, Nizard C. Hormesis-based anti-aging products: a case study of a novel cosmetic. Dose Response. 2013;11(1):99-108.

[20] Oh SJ, Kim K, Lim CJ. Suppressive properties of ginsenoside Rb2, a protopanaxadiol-type ginseng saponin, on reactive oxygen species and matrix metalloproteinase-2 in UV-B-irradiated human dermal keratinocytes. Biosci Biotechnol Biochem. 2015;79(7): 1075-81.

[21] Lim CJ, Choi WY, Jung HJ. Stereoselective skin anti-photoaging properties of ginsenoside Rg3 in UV-B-irradiated keratinocytes. Biol Pharm Bull. 2014;37(10):1583-90.

[22] Oh SJ, Lee S, Choi WY, Lim CJ. Skin anti-photoaging properties of ginsenoside Rh2 epimers in UV-B-irradiated human keratinocyte cells. J Biosci. 2014;39(4):673-82.

[23] Kim YG, Sumiyoshi M, Sakanaka M, Kimura Y. Effects of ginseng saponins isolated from red ginseng on ultraviolet B-induced skin aging in hairless mice. Eur J Pharmacol. 2009;602(1):148-56.

[24] Lee EH, Cho SY, Kim SJ, Shin ES, Chang HK, Kim DH, et al. Ginsenoside F1 protects human HaCaT keratinocytes from ultraviolet-B-induced apoptosis by maintaining constant levels of Bcl-2. J Invest Dermatol. 2003;121(3):607-13.

[25] Pham QL, Jang HJ, Kim KB. Antiwrinkle effect of fermented black ginseng on human fibroblasts. Int J Mol Med. 2017;39(3):681-6.

[26] Hwang E, Park SY, Yin CS, Kim HT, Kim YM, Yi TH. Antiaging effects of the mixture of *Panax ginseng* and *Crataegus pinnatifida* in human dermal fibroblasts and healthy human skin. J Ginseng Res. 2017;41(1):69-77.

[27] Lee GY, Park KG, Namgoong S, Han SK, Jeong SH, Dhong ES, et al. Effects of *Panax ginseng* extract on human dermal fibroblast proliferation and collagen synthesis. Int Wound J. 2016;13 Suppl 1:42-6.

[28] Lee J, Jung E, Lee J, Huh S, Kim J, Park M, et al. *Panax ginseng* induces human Type I collagen synthesis through activation of Smad signaling. J Ethnopharmacol. 2007;109(1):29-34.

[29] Papakonstantinou E, Roth M, Karakiulakis G. Hyaluronic acid: A key molecule in skin aging. Dermatoendocrinol. 2012;4(3):253-8.

[30] Kim S, Kang BY, Cho SY, Sung DS, Chang HK, Yeom MH, et al. Compound K induces expression of hyaluronan synthase 2 gene in transformed human keratinocytes and increases hyaluronan in hairless mouse skin. Biochem Biophys Res Commun. 2004;316(2):348-55.

[31] Chan L, Cook DK. Female pattern hair loss. Aust J Gen Pract. 2018;47(7): 459-64.

[32] Tanaka Y, Aso T, Ono J, Hosoi R, Kaneko T. Androgenetic Alopecia Treatment in Asian Men. J Clin Aesthet Dermatol. 2018;11(7):32-5.

[33] Kaufman KD, Olsen EA, Whiting D, Savin R, DeVillez R, Bergfeld W, et al. Finasteride in the treatment of men with androgenetic alopecia. Finasteride Male Pattern Hair Loss Study Group. J Am Acad Dermatol. 1998;39(4 Pt 1):578-89.

[34] Asada Y, Sonoda T, Ojiro M, Kurata S, Sato T, Ezaki T, et al. 5 alpha-reductase type 2 is constitutively expressed in the dermal papilla and connective tissue sheath of the hair follicle in vivo but not during culture in vitro. J Clin Endocrinol Metab. 2001;86(6):2875-80.

[35] Murata K, Takeshita F, Samukawa K, Tani T, Matsuda H. Effects of ginseng rhizome and ginsenoside Ro on testosterone 5alpha-reductase and hair

re-growth in testosterone-treated mice. Phytother Res. 2012;26(1):48-53.

[36] Shin DH, Cha YJ, Yang KE, Jang IS, Son CG, Kim BH, et al. Ginsenoside Rg3 up-regulates the expression of vascular endothelial growth factor in human dermal papilla cells and mouse hair follicles. Phytother Res. 2014;28(7): 1088-95.

[37] Truong VL, Bak MJ, Lee C, Jun M, Jeong WS. Hair Regenerative Mechanisms of Red Ginseng Oil and Its Major Components in the Testosterone-Induced Delay of Anagen Entry in C57BL/6 Mice. Molecules. 2017;22(9).

[38] Inui S, Itami S. Molecular basis of androgenetic alopecia: From androgen to paracrine mediators through dermal papilla. J Dermatol Sci. 2011;61(1):1-6.

[39] Majeed F, Malik FZ, Ahmed Z, Afreen A, Afzal MN, Khalid N. Ginseng phytochemicals as therapeutics in oncology: Recent perspectives. Biomed Pharmacother. 2018;100:52-63.

[40] Johnson KE, Wilgus TA. Vascular Endothelial Growth Factor and Angiogenesis in the Regulation of Cutaneous Wound Repair. Adv Wound Care (New Rochelle). 2014;3(10): 647-61.

[41] Mattioli M, Barboni B, Turriani M, Galeati G, Zannoni A, Castellani G, et al. Follicle activation involves vascular endothelial growth factor production and increased blood vessel extension. Biol Reprod. 2001;65(4):1014-9.

[42] Li W, Man XY, Li CM, Chen JQ, Zhou J, Cai SQ, et al. VEGF induces proliferation of human hair follicle dermal papilla cells through VEGFR-2-mediated activation of ERK. Exp Cell Res. 2012;318(14):1633-40.

[43] Shin HS, Park SY, Hwang ES, Lee DG, Song HG, Mavlonov GT, et al. The inductive effect of ginsenoside F2

on hair growth by altering the WNT signal pathway in telogen mouse skin. European journal of pharmacology. 2014;730:82-9.

[44] Han JH, Kwon OS, Chung JH, Cho KH, Eun HC, Kim KH. Effect of minoxidil on proliferation and apoptosis in dermal papilla cells of human hair follicle. J Dermatol Sci. 2004;34(2):91-8.

[45] Lee NE, Park SD, Hwang H, Choi SH, Lee RM, Nam SM, et al. Effects of a gintonin-enriched fraction on hair growth: an in vitro and in vivo study. J Ginseng Res. 2020;44(1):168-77.

[46] Lindner G, Botchkarev VA, Botchkareva NV, Ling G, van der Veen C, Paus R. Analysis of apoptosis during hair follicle regression (catagen). Am J Pathol. 1997;151(6):1601-17.

[47] Muller-Rover S, Rossiter H, Lindner G, Peters EM, Kupper TS, Paus R. Hair follicle apoptosis and Bcl-2. J Investig Dermatol Symp Proc. 1999;4(3):272-7.

[48] Muller-Rover S, Rossiter H, Paus R, Handjiski B, Peters EM, Murphy JE, et al. Overexpression of Bcl-2 protects from ultraviolet B-induced apoptosis but promotes hair follicle regression and chemotherapy-induced alopecia. Am J Pathol. 2000;156(4):1395-405.

[49] Park S, Shin WS, Ho J. Fructus *Panax ginseng* extract promotes hair regeneration in C57BL/6 mice. J Ethnopharmacol. 2011;138(2):340-4.

[50] Andl T, Reddy ST, Gaddapara T, Millar SE. WNT signals are required for the initiation of hair follicle development. Dev Cell. 2002;2(5): 643-53.

[51] Kretzschmar K, Cottle DL, Schweiger PJ, Watt FM. The Androgen Receptor Antagonizes Wnt/beta-Catenin Signaling in Epidermal Stem Cells. J Invest Dermatol. 2015;135(11): 2753-63.

[52] Kretzschmar K, Clevers H. Wnt/beta-catenin signaling in adult mammalian epithelial stem cells. Dev Biol. 2017;428(2):273-82.

[53] Huelsken J, Vogel R, Erdmann B, Cotsarelis G, Birchmeier W. beta-Catenin controls hair follicle morphogenesis and stem cell differentiation in the skin. Cell. 2001;105(4):533-45.

[54] Kishimoto J, Burgeson RE, Morgan BA. Wnt signaling maintains the hair-inducing activity of the dermal papilla. Genes Dev. 2000;14(10):1181-5.

[55] Sato N, Leopold PL, Crystal RG. Effect of adenovirus-mediated expression of Sonic hedgehog gene on hair regrowth in mice with chemotherapy-induced alopecia. J Natl Cancer Inst. 2001;93(24):1858-64.

[56] Wang LC, Liu ZY, Gambardella L, Delacour A, Shapiro R, Yang J, et al. Regular articles: conditional disruption of hedgehog signaling pathway defines its critical role in hair development and regeneration. J Invest Dermatol. 2000;114(5):901-8.

[57] Foitzik K, Lindner G, Mueller-Roever S, Maurer M, Botchkareva N, Botchkarev V, et al. Control of murine hair follicle regression (catagen) by TGF-beta1 in vivo. FASEB J. 2000;14(5):752-60.

[58] Peters EM, Hansen MG, Overall RW, Nakamura M, Pertile P, Klapp BF, et al. Control of human hair growth by neurotrophins: brain-derived neurotrophic factor inhibits hair shaft elongation, induces catagen, and stimulates follicular transforming growth factor beta2 expression. J Invest Dermatol. 2005;124(4):675-85.

[59] Shin H, Yoo HG, Inui S, Itami S, Kim IG, Cho AR, et al. Induction of transforming growth factor-beta 1 by androgen is mediated by reactive oxygen species in hair follicle dermal papilla cells. BMB Rep. 2013;46(9):460-4.

[60] Kim YG, Sumiyoshi M, Kawahira K, Sakanaka M, Kimura Y. Effects of Red Ginseng extract on ultraviolet B-irradiated skin change in C57BL mice. Phytother Res. 2008;22(11):1423-7.

[61] Li Z, Ryu SW, Lee J, Choi K, Kim S, Choi C. Protopanaxatirol type ginsenoside Re promotes cyclic growth of hair follicles via inhibiting transforming growth factor beta signaling cascades. Biochem Biophys Res Commun. 2016;470(4):924-9.

[62] Chang JW, Park KH, Hwang HS, Shin YS, Oh YT, Kim CH. Protective effects of Korean red ginseng against radiation-induced apoptosis in human HaCaT keratinocytes. J Radiat Res. 2014;55(2):245-56.

[63] Matsuda H, Yamazaki M, Asanuma Y, Kubo M. Promotion of hair growth by ginseng radix on cultured mouse vibrissal hair follicles. Phytother Res. 2003;17(7):797-800.

[64] Lee Y, Kim SN, Hong YD, Park BC, Na Y. Panax ginseng extract antagonizes the effect of DKK1-induced catagen-like changes of hair follicles. Int J Mol Med. 2017;40(4):1194-200.

[65] Danilenko DM, Ring BD, Pierce GF. Growth factors and cytokines in hair follicle development and cycling: recent insights from animal models and the potentials for clinical therapy. Molecular medicine today. 1996;2(11):460-7.

[66] Hoffmann R, Eicheler W, Huth A, Wenzel E, Happle R. Cytokines and growth factors influence hair growth in vitro. Possible implications for the pathogenesis and treatment of alopecia areata. Archives of dermatological research. 1996;288(3):153-6.

[67] Ito T, Ito N, Saatoff M, Hashizume H, Fukamizu H,

Nickoloff BJ, et al. Maintenance of hair follicle immune privilege is linked to prevention of NK cell attack. J Invest Dermatol. 2008;128(5):1196-206.

[68] Paus R, Ito N, Takigawa M, Ito T. The hair follicle and immune privilege. J Investig Dermatol Symp Proc. 2003;8(2):188-94.

[69] Christoph T, Muller-Rover S, Audring H, Tobin DJ, Hermes B, Cotsarelis G, et al. The human hair follicle immune system: cellular composition and immune privilege. The British journal of dermatology. 2000;142(5):862-73.

[70] Hu J, Batth IS, Xia X, Li S. Regulation of NKG2D(+)CD8(+) T-cell-mediated antitumor immune surveillance: Identification of a novel CD28 activation-mediated, STAT3 phosphorylation-dependent mechanism. Oncoimmunology. 2016;5(12):e1252012.

[71] Triyangkulsri K, Suchonwanit P. Role of janus kinase inhibitors in the treatment of alopecia areata. Drug Des Devel Ther. 2018;12:2323-35.

[72] Ismail FF, Sinclair R. JAK inhibition in the treatment of alopecia areata - a promising new dawn? Expert review of clinical pharmacology. 2020;13(1):43-51.

[73] Iorizzo M, Tosti A. Emerging drugs for alopecia areata: JAK inhibitors. Expert opinion on emerging drugs. 2018;23(1):77-81.

[74] Yu Q, Zeng KW, Ma XL, Jiang Y, Tu PF, Wang XM. Ginsenoside Rk1 suppresses pro-inflammatory responses in lipopolysaccharide-stimulated RAW264.7 cells by inhibiting the Jak2/Stat3 pathway. Chin J Nat Med. 2017;15(10):751-7.

[75] Han S, Jeong AJ, Yang H, Bin Kang K, Lee H, Yi EH, et al. Ginsenoside 20(S)-Rh2 exerts anti-cancer activity through targeting IL-6-induced JAK2/STAT3 pathway in human colorectal cancer cells. Journal of ethnopharmacology. 2016;194:83-90.

[76] Guttman-Yassky E, Nia JK, Hashim PW, Mansouri Y, Alia E, Taliercio M, et al. Efficacy and safety of secukinumab treatment in adults with extensive alopecia areata. Arch Dermatol Res. 2018;310(8):607-14.

[77] Wei Y, Huyghues-Despointes BM, Tsai J, Scholtz JM. NMR study and molecular dynamics simulations of optimized beta-hairpin fragments of protein G. Proteins. 2007;69(2):285-96.

www.ingramcontent.com/pod-product-compliance
Lightning Source LLC
Chambersburg PA
CBHW081235190326
41458CB00016B/5785